LEVEL 1

Introduction to Health & Social Care and Children & Young People's Settings

Corinne Barker and Emma Ward

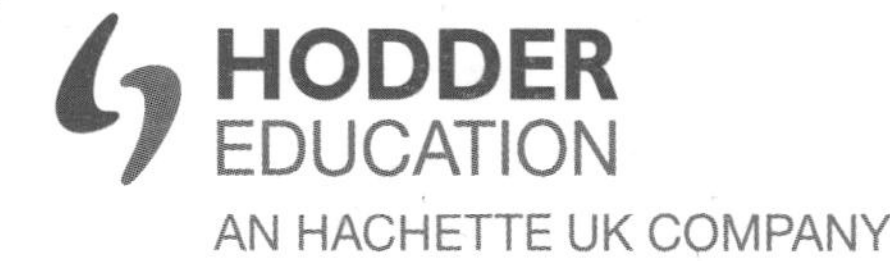

Orders: please contact Bookpoint Ltd, 130 Milton Park, Abingdon, Oxon OX14 4SB. Telephone: (44) 01235 827720. Fax: (44) 01235 400454. Lines are open from 9.00 to 5.00, Monday to Saturday, with a 24-hour message answering service. You can also order through our website www.hoddereducation.co.uk

If you have any comments to make about this, or any of our other titles, please send them to educationenquiries@hodder.co.uk

British Library Cataloguing in Publication Data

A catalogue record for this title is available from the British Library

ISBN: 978 1471 83017 4

This Edition Published 2014

Impression number 10 9 8 7 6 5 4 3 2 1

Year 2017, 2016, 2015, 2014

Typeset by Integra Software Services Pvt. Ltd., Pondicherry, India.

Printed in Italy.

Contents

Acknowledgements

We would like to thank colleagues and students at Wakefield College who have contributed ideas and taken such an interest in the writing of this textbook.

Thank you to our ever-understanding families and to our children, Stevie, Jake, Eva and Ben, who constantly inspire us!

We would also like to thank the editorial team at Hodder Education, in particular, Stephen Halder, publisher; Sebastian Rydberg, desk editor; and Annette McFadyen, freelance copy-editor, for their support.

Corinne and Emma

Picture credits

The publishers would like to thank all the staff, children and families at Vanessa Nursery School, Ark Alpha Nursery, Godington Day Nursery and Kate Greenaway Nursery School and Children's Centre for their help with many of the photographs, taken by Jules Selmes, Andrew Callaghan, and Justin O'Hanlon. A special thanks to Michele Barrett and Julie Breading for all their assistance with the organisation of the photo-shoots.

Every effort has been made to trace the copyright holders of material reproduced here. The authors and publishers would like to thank the following for permission to reproduce copyright illustrations:

p.viii © tsuppyinny – Fotolia.com; p.2 © pix4U – Fotolia.com; p.3 © Lisa F. Young – Fotolia.com; p.4 © spotmatikphoto – Fotolia.com; p.5 © Hunor Kristo – Forolia.com; p.8 l © Trish23 – Fotolia.com, r © Monkey Business – Fotolia.com; p.9 © CandyBox Images – Fotolia.com; p.11 t © Justin O'Hanlon b © Bubbles Photolibrary / Alamy; p.16 © Jules Selmes; p.18 t © Purestock / Alamy, b © Blend Images / Alamy; p.19 © contrastwerkstatt – Fotolia.com; p.22 © Juice Images / Alamy; p.23 t © Jules Selmes, bl © Francisco Martinez / Alamy, br © migstock / Alamy; p.24 © Blend Images / Alamy; p.25 l © Courtesy of Childline, a service provided by NSPCC, r © Courtesy of NSPCC; p.26 © diego cervo – Fotolia.com; p.27 © Alin a Vincent Photography, LLC – Getty Images; p.28 © Rido – Fotolia.com; p.32 tl © Rich Legg – Getty Images, tr © Purestock / Alamy, m Jules Selmes, b © Alexander Raths – Fotolia.com; p.33 © sepy – Fotolia.com; p.35 t © imageBROKER / Alamy, b © Image Source / Alamy; p.36 t © nyul – Fotolia.com, b © Monkey Business – Fotolia.com; p.37 tl © Monkey Business – Fotolia.com, tr © Monkey Business – Fotolia.com, bl © DragonImages – Fotolia.com, br © Blend Images / Alamy; p.38 t © Jules Selmes, bl © Jeanette Dietl – Fotolia.com, br

© JPC-PROD – Fotolia; p.40 t © Halfpoint – Fotolia.com, b © Jules Selmes; p.41 l © goodluz – Fotolia.com, r © IMAGEMORE Co., Ltd. / Alamy; p.46 © Ian Shaw / Alamy; p.47 © Golden Pixels LLC / Alamy; p.48 t © WavebreakmediaMicro - Fotolia.com, b © Bubbles Photolibrary / Alamy; p.50 © Franz Pfluegl – Fotolia.com; p.51 © motto – Fotolia.com; p.54 © RTimages – Fotolia.com; p.55 t © MBI / Alamy, bl © stocksolutions – Fotolia.com, br © Monika Wisniewska – Fotolia.com; p.56 t © Arcaid Images / Alamy, b © Todd Bannor / Alamy; p.57 © BSIP SA / Alamy; p.58 © Image Source / Alamy; p.60 t © Tina Chang/ Corbis, b © cobraphoto – Fotolia.com; p.62 © doble.d – Fotolia.com; p.67 © amana images inc. / Alamy; p.68 © Jules Selmes; p.69 © Vstock LLC – Getty Images; p.71 © Jules Selmes; p.72 © Jupiterimages – Stockbyte – Thinkstock; p.73 © michaeljung - Fotolia.com; p.77 © wckiw – Fotolia.com; p.80 © volff – Fotolia.com; p.84 © Blend Images / Alamy; p.87 © Lsantilli – Fotolia.com; p.89 © Barking Dog Art; p.90 © micromonkey – Fotolia.com; p.91 © witthaya – Fotolia.com; p.93 © Rob Melynchuk – Getty Images; p.96 © ivolodina -Fotolia.com; p.97 © Elena Stepanova – Fotolia.com; p.98 © SerrNovik – Fotolia.com; p.99 © Jules Selmes; p.100 © Photographee.eu – Fotolia.com; p.102 © Jules Selmes; p.103 t ©Jules Selmes, m © Valua Vitaly – Fotolia.com, b © Lisa F. Young – Fotolia.com; p.113 © Monkey Business – Fotolia.com; p.116 © Glenda Powers – Fotolia.com; p.119 © medbeam – Fotolia.com; p.120 © singkham – Fotolia.com; p.121 l © apops – Fotolia.com, r © william87 – Fotolia.com; p.129 © Dan Race – Fotolia.com; p.130 l © Steve Vidler / Alamy, r © David R. Frazier Photolibrary, Inc. / Alamy; p.132 © mezzotint_fotolia – Fotolia.com; p.133 © Kiko Jimenez – Fotolia.com; p.134 © Grafvision – Fotolia.com; p.136 © Angela Hampton Picture Library / Alamy; p.139 © Kalim – Fotolia.com; p.142 © Photographee.eu - Fotolia.com; p.144 © giideon – Fotolia.com; p.150 © lamma – Fotolia.com; p.151 © Andrey Bandurenko – Fotolia.com; p.152 © davizro photography – Fotolia.com; p.158 © Africa Studio – Fotolia.com; p.159 © Photononstop / Alamy; p.162 © Lydia Young; p.163 © Crown copyright material as reproduced with the permission of the controller of HMSO and the Queen's Printers of Scotland; p.167 © Jules Selmes; p.168 t © Jules Selmes, b © Andrew Callaghan; p.170 © Andrew Callaghan.

How to use this book

Make real progress with this Introduction to Health & Social Care and Children & Young People's Settings! This book guides you through the 7 mandatory units and 11 optional units exploring safeguarding and communication to healthy eating, and growth and development. Each unit includes headings clearly matched to the specification and links to assessment criteria, as well as an array of activities to help you generate evidence.

Key features of the book

Understand the requirements of the new qualification with headings linked to learning outcomes and assessment criteria

What you will learn in this unit

You will gain an understanding of:

- The ways that children learn.

Prepare for what you are going to cover in the unit

Observation

They may also enjoy planting seeds to find out how vegetables and flowers grow.

1 For example, children could pretend to be a solider or a pirate or act out a story, perhaps using small characters or animals.

Guidance on specific things to observe and look out for, and how best to incorporate observation as part of practice

Information box

Children may experiment by dropping objects into water to see if they float or sink to the bottom. Bath time is a time when children will often experiment with bubbles or floating toys.

Remember key points and useful information

Important words

Senses – Touch, smell, taste, sight and hearing: used to make sense of the world around us

Understand important terms

Task!

Mai is going to the supermarket with her Grandma.
In pairs discuss and write down the opportunities that Mai might have to investigate the environment using each of her senses.

Short tasks to help you test your understanding

Safety warning

It is important to look at the environment and where possible reduce the chance of a child or adult being injured or harmed.

Highlight any important points regarding health and safety

Example!

Aadi will enjoy watching Mai completing a jigsaw, but will learn more about shape and size by trying to fit the pieces of jigsaw together by himself.

Short examples and scenarios help you explore key issues and relate theory to practice

Assessment task 1.1

1 Describe the boundaries and rules used in your setting to promote positive behaviour, and explain why staff should apply these consistently and fairly.

An activity linked to assessment criteria to help you generate evidence

Assessment guidance

Promoting children's positive behaviour

Check that you know what the policies and procedures are for promoting positive behaviour in your work setting.

Important guidance and tips to help you prepare for assessment

Summary

Check that you know what the policies and procedures are for promoting positive behaviour in your work setting:

Recap the key issues covered in the unit

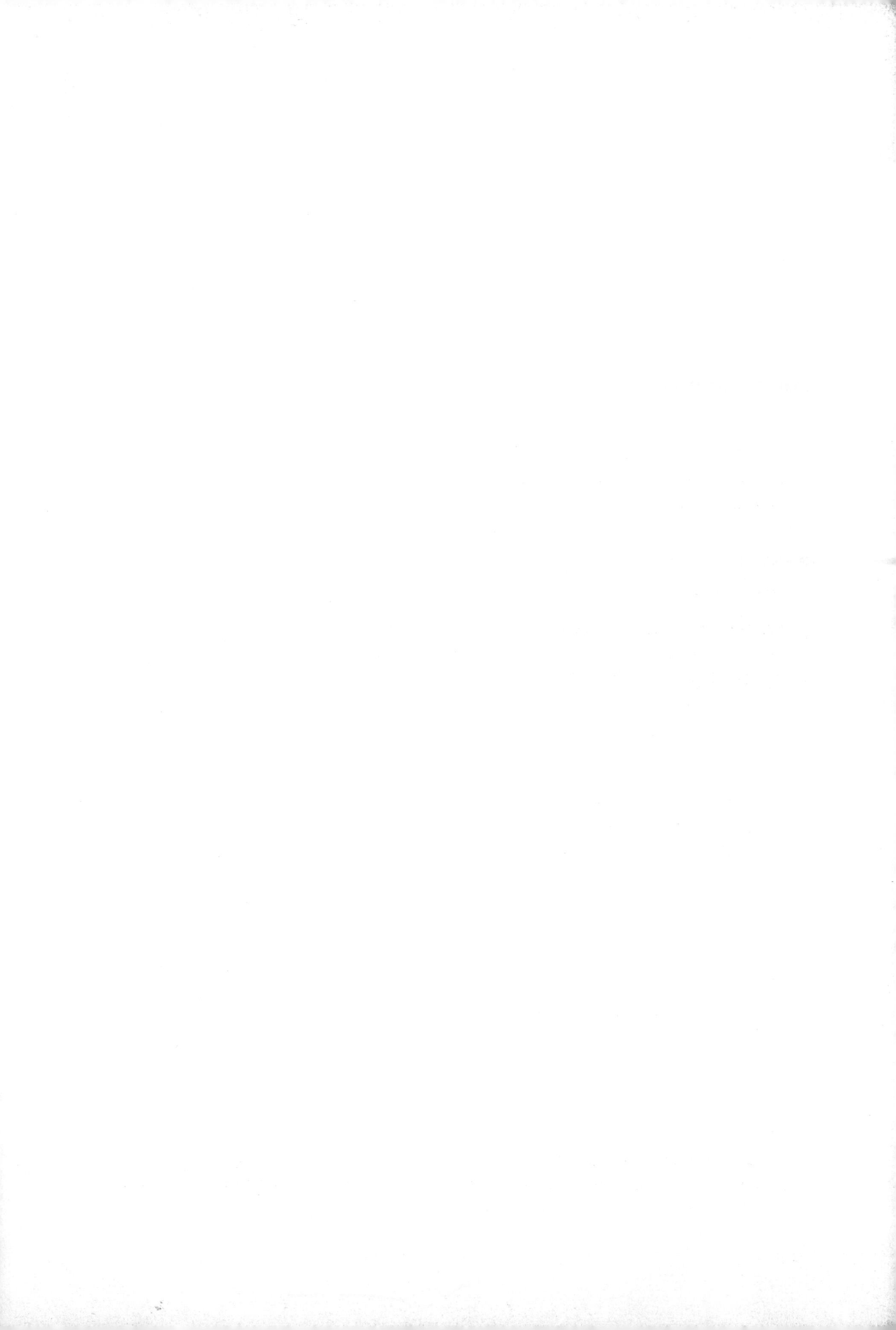

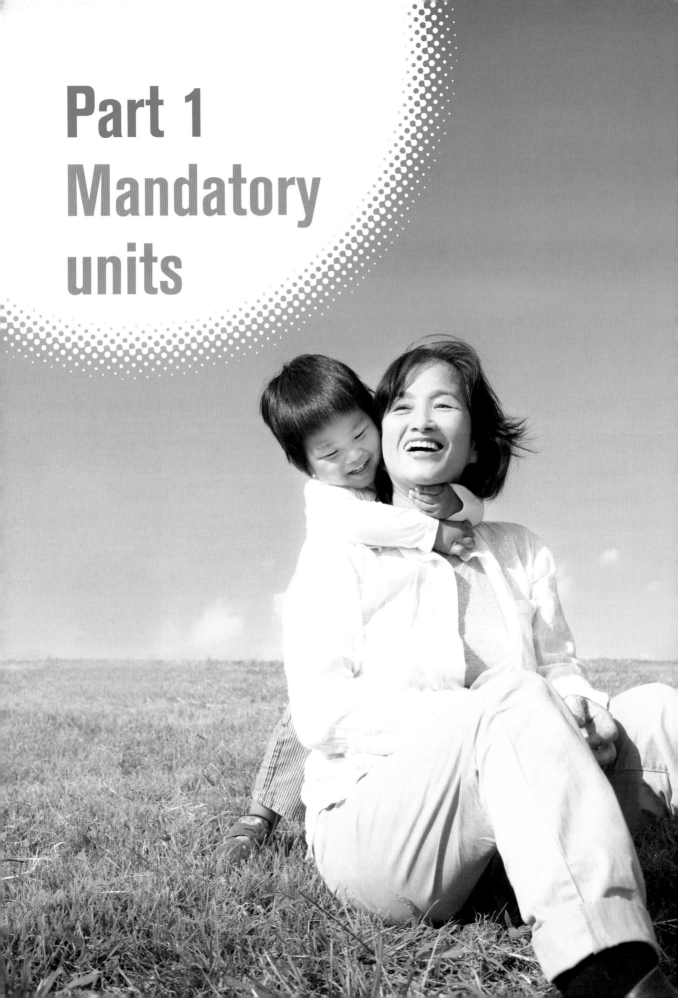

Part 1 Mandatory units

Chapter 1

Intro MU 1.1 Understand the range of service provision and roles within health and social care (adults and children and young people), early years and childcare

What you will learn in this unit

- The range of service provision available in health care, social care and childcare.
- The difference between statutory and independent service provision.
- The different job roles within health care, social care and childcare and the skills required to carry out these roles.
- Progression routes for employment in health care, social care and childcare.

Important words

Employment – A job that you are paid to do

Service provision – These are services that are available for people to use

Service user – Someone who uses the service

The range of service provision in health care, social care and childcare

1.1 1.2 1.3 Identify the range of service provision, outline the purpose of the service provision, and give examples of who would access different types of service provision

Types and purpose of service provision

There are many different types of health care, social care and childcare available for people to use. Care services can be statutory, independent or informal and can include the following types of service provision, as listed in the table below.

Type of service provision 1.1	Purpose of the provision 1.2	Who may access the service provision 1.3
Day care for adults	• Many care homes for adults with a disability have closed down • Adults may want to continue to live in their own home • Provides social activities for adults with a disability	Adults with a disability who need day-to-day support
Hospital accident and emergency department	• To provide emergency treatment when a person suddenly becomes seriously ill • If someone has a dangerous or life-threatening accident	Everyone
Residential services for children and young people (foster care)	• Provides safe care for children and young people who cannot live with their own family	Children and young people
Tele care, e.g. 999 emergency service, Childline, Samaritans	• Provides medical advice to people who phone asking for help • Supports people in times of crisis	Everyone in need of advice and support People who do not know where to go to get help

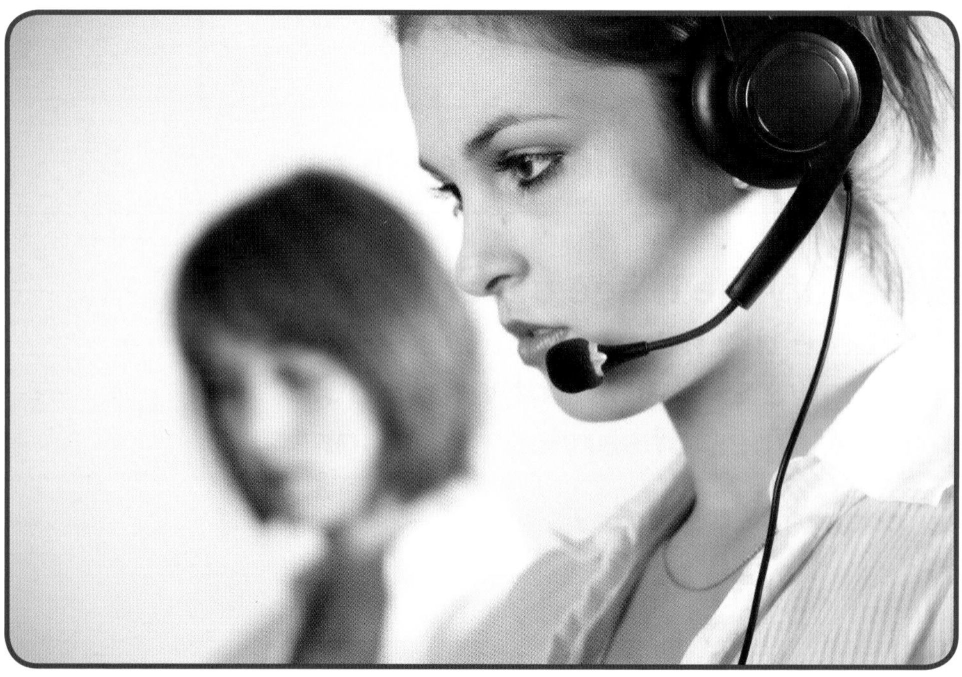

Figure 1.1

Type of service provision 1.1	Purpose of the provision 1.2	Who may access the service provision 1.3
Community-based services, e.g. home help, community nurses, meals service	• Provides care for people who need support to live in their own home • Provides medical care for people who are ill but not staying in hospital • Helps to provide for care needs (dressing, bathing, providing meals)	Older aged adults Anyone with a disability or additional need
Day nurseries	• Provides care and education for young children 0–5 years • Needed by working families during working hours • Allows children to socialise with others	Children and their families
Doctor's (GP's) surgery	• Diagnoses and treats illness and gives prescriptions for medication • Gives health care advice • Organises support groups	Everyone
Complementary therapies	Can be used instead of or alongside medical treatment, e.g. homeopathy, reflexology, massage	Everyone

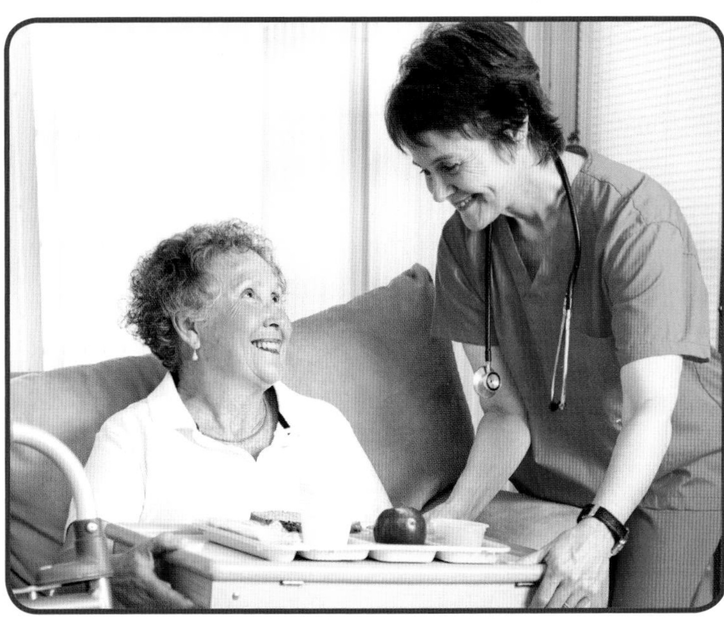

Figure 1.2

Type of service provision 1.1	Purpose of the provision 1.2	Who may access the service provision 1.3
Community pharmacy (chemist)	• Gives out prescription medicine • Sells non-prescription medicine and first aid supplies • Offers healthcare support and advice, e.g. stopping smoking, contraception advice	Everyone
Substance misuse services	• Supports the safety of drug users (needle exchange) • Offers counselling and rehabilitation services	People with addictions
Residential care home	• Provides full-time care for older aged adults who are no longer able to care for themselves • Older aged adults can receive short-term care, e.g. to give their main carer a break	Older aged adults

Table 1.1 Types and purpose of service provision, and who may use the provision

Task!

What services might these people use?

- A child who has broken their arm when playing
- An older aged adult living in their own home who finds it difficult to cook their own meals
- A young person with an addiction

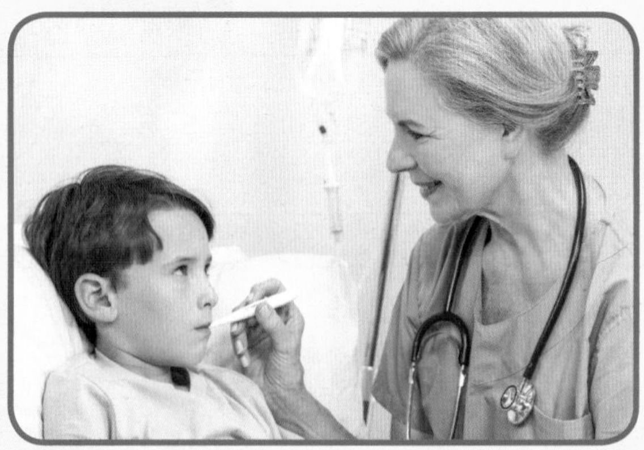

Figure 1.3

Assessment task 1.1 1.2 1.3

Identify at least two different providers of health, social or childcare services in your own local area. For each one, explain the purpose of the provision and give an example of who would access the service. You can use a table like the one below:

Type of service	Purpose of service	Example of user of service

1.4 Outline the difference between statutory and independent service provision

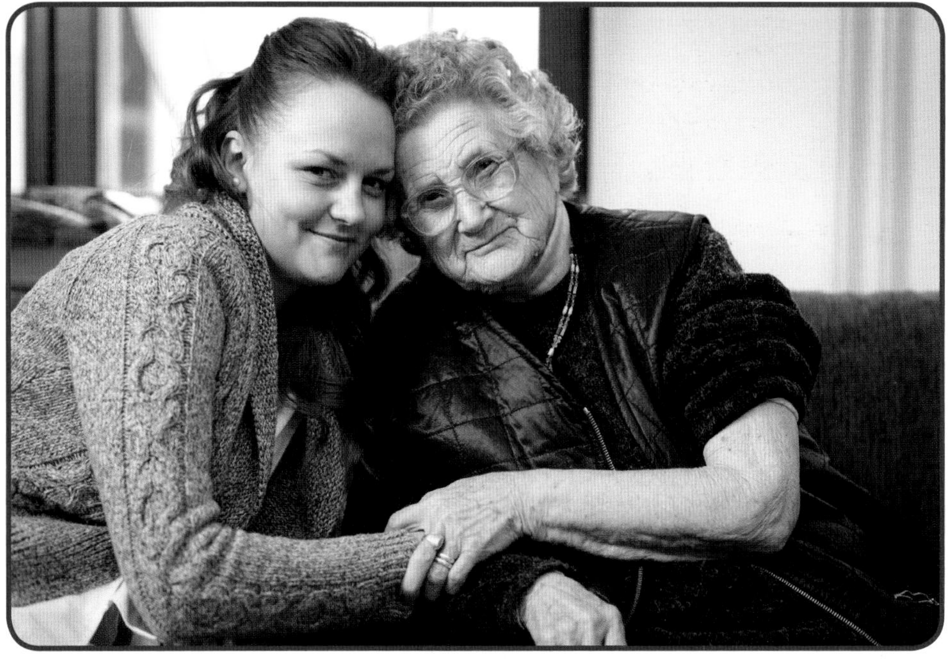

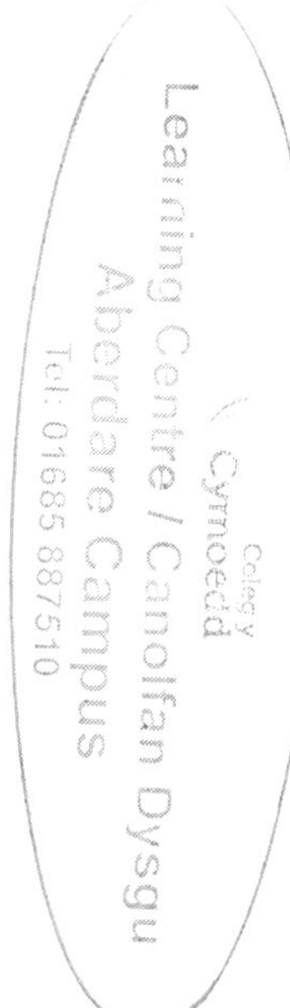

Figure 1.4

A **statutory service** should be available to everyone by law.

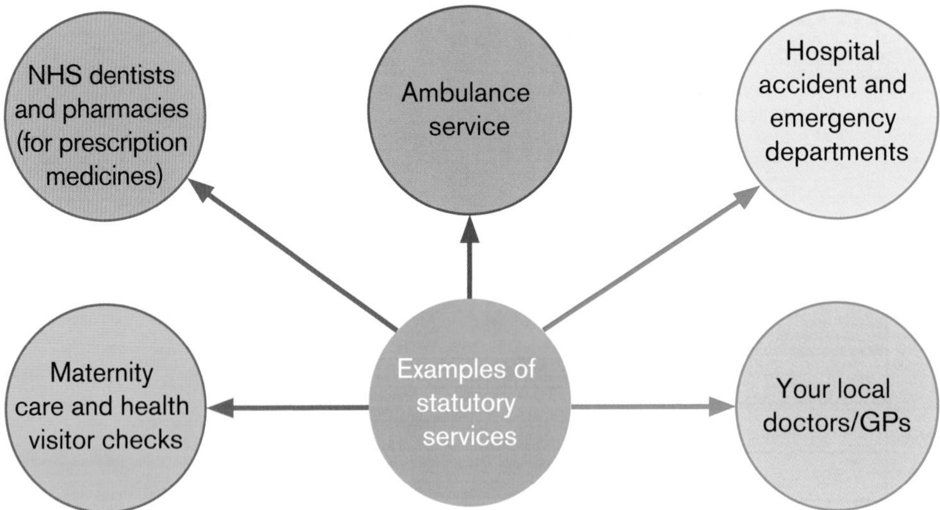

Figure 1.5 Examples of statutory services

An **independent service** does not have to be provided by law but can be provided by people or companies who charge for the service. A **voluntary** service is provided by people who do not get paid and do not expect payment from the people who need help.

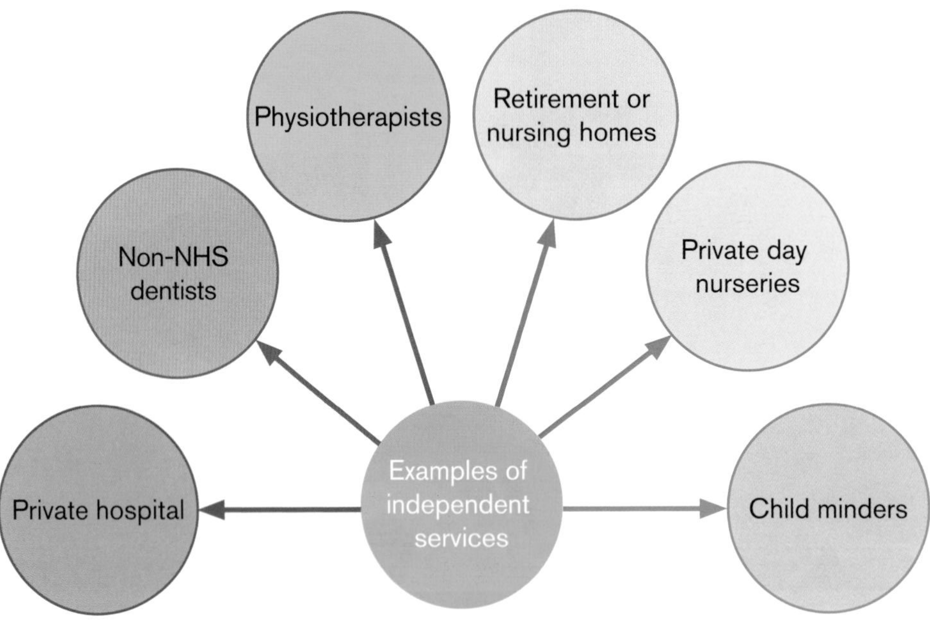

Figure 1.6 Examples of independent services

1.5 Outline how informal care contributes to provision

Informal care may be given by family, friends, neighbours or members of the local community. This type of care may be provided for a short time; for example, if someone is recovering from an illness and cannot yet meet their own care needs (washing, cooking and cleaning), a neighbour may offer to help until they are able to do these things for themselves.

Informal care may also be long term, for example, a family member looking after an older aged parent so that they do not have to go into a care home. Informal care is very important within communities as it means that people do not always have to use statutory services, such as hospitals, which can sometimes become too full. It also means that anyone who cannot afford to pay for independent services can still be cared for.

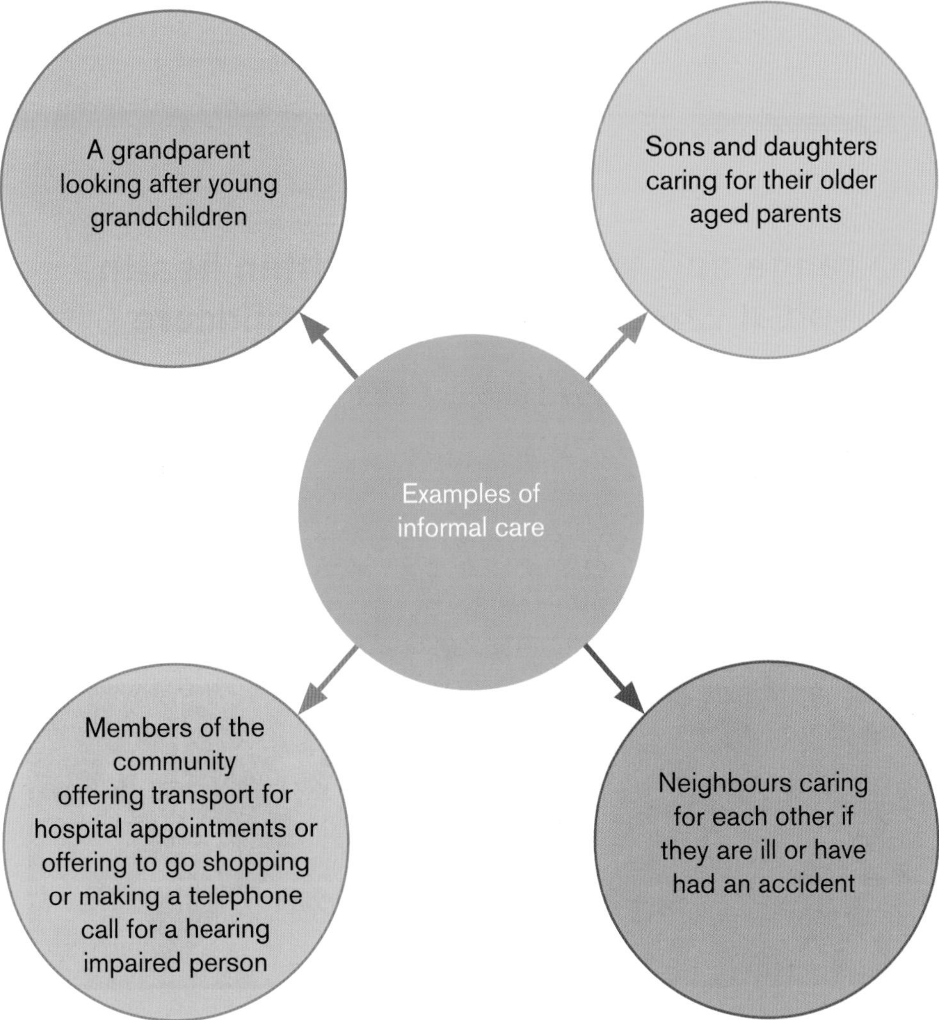

Figure 1.7 Examples of informal care

Task!

What do you think?

A neighbour goes shopping for an older aged person. Is this a statutory service? Yes/No

You have an appointment with your local doctor. Is this a statutory service? Yes/No

An alcohol-dependent adult phones a helpline for help. Is this an informal service? Yes/No

Assessment task 1.4 1.5

Make a leaflet for service users that explains about statutory services and independent services and the differences between these services.

In your leaflet, give information about informal care and say how this can help people.

The range and scope of roles within health and social care, early years and childcare

2.1 Job roles within health care, social care and childcare

There are many job roles within health and social care and childcare. Some of these job roles are needed in health, social and childcare, for example, receptionist, cleaner or health visitor. Other job roles are only needed in one of these types of service; for example, a midwife or doctor would only work within health care services.

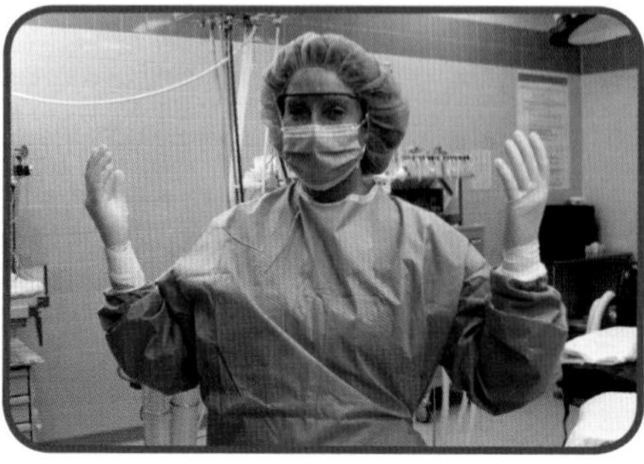

Figure 1.8 A doctor

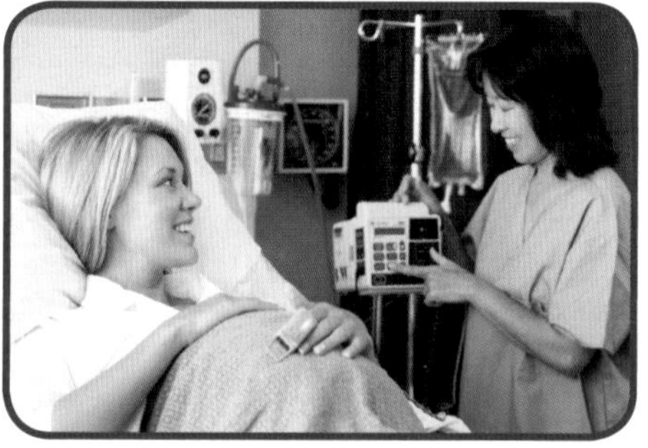

Figure 1.9 A midwife caring for a patient

Assessment task 2.1

Research or discuss the list of job roles below and sort them into the correct service. Remember – some job roles may fit into more than one service.

- Domestic assistant
- Health visitor
- Midwife
- Physiotherapist
- Play therapist
- Occupational therapist
- Receptionist
- Social worker
- Community care worker
- Childcare worker

Health care	Social care	Childcare

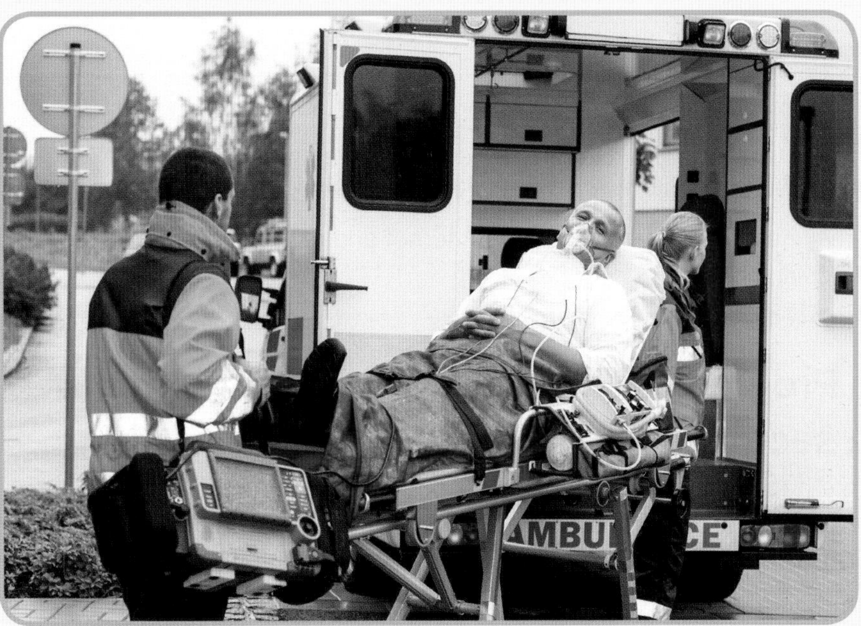

Figure 1.10 Paramedics at work

2.2 Knowledge and skills required to work in health, social care and childcare

Every job role has its own set of roles and responsibilities. People need to have the correct qualifications and skills to be able to do certain jobs. For example:

A nurse needs to have a nursing qualification before they are allowed to care for people; however, to do the job well they also need to be kind, caring, want to help others and have good communication skills.

A nursery worker in a day nursery will need to have a childcare qualification, but they will also need to follow all the policies and procedures carefully, be very reliable and show patience and understanding towards the children.

A doctor spends many years at university learning how to diagnose and treat illness. A doctor will need to be very interested in the health of others and be able to take responsibility for their care and treatment. Doctors need to be able to read and understand information so that they are aware of all the new treatments that become available.

Assessment task 2.3

Choose two other job roles from the lists above and research the knowledge and skills required to work in these jobs.

(It may help you if you look on the internet and read job descriptions for particular job roles.)

2.3 Progression routes for workers within the sector

Once a health, social or childcare worker has qualified to do a job, they may decide that they would like to progress within the service and take on a different role with more responsibility or challenges.

Example!

Josh, a nursery worker, looks at what the nursery manager does every day and decides that in the future, when he has more experience, that will be the job role he would like to do. It is important that Josh finds out about any further qualifications he will need, in order to work towards his goal of becoming a nursery manager.

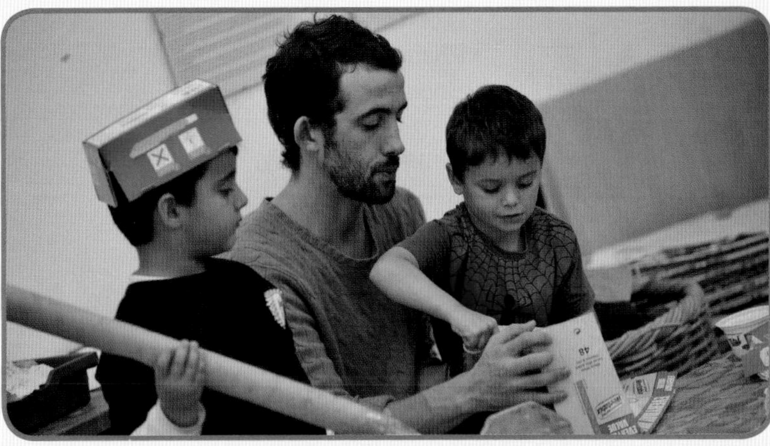

Figure 1.11

Ruby has worked as a domestic assistant on a children's ward in a hospital for ten years. She has always observed the hospital play therapist who works with sick children and thought this would be her dream job. Her children have now all left home and she feels it is the right time to further her career and train as a play therapist. Ruby did not get many qualifications at school so she is going to college in the evening to get the qualifications she needs to apply for this training.

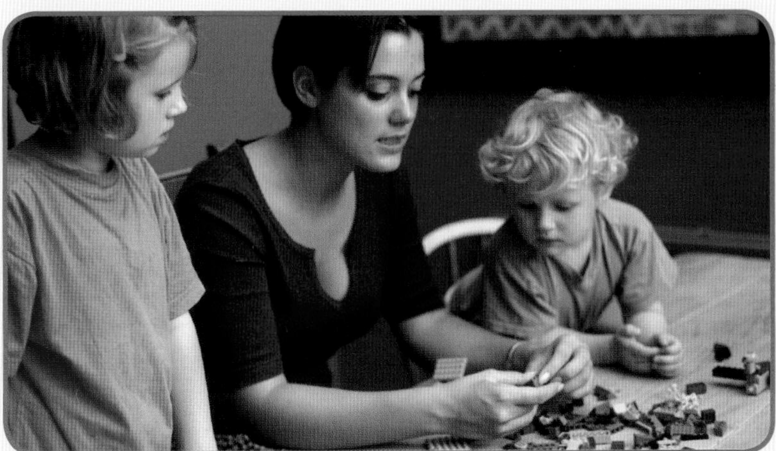

Figure 1.12

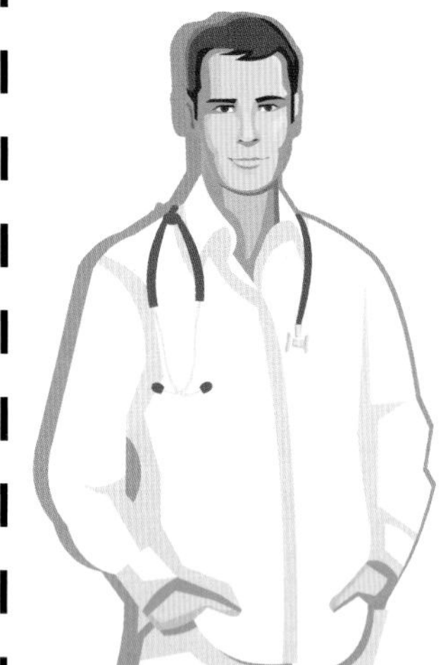

Doctors wanted!
Golden opportunity to enhance your skills and career at
Sunnyvale Health Centre
• Dentists
• Dieticians
• Pharmacists
• Social workers
(Competitive salary)

Figure 1.13 Example of a job advertisement

Assessment task 2.3

Iram works in a children's centre and enjoys her job; however, Iram has always been interested in becoming a midwife.

Outline the progression route that Iram must take to become a midwife.

(It may help you to research midwifery courses available at university and the qualifications needed to apply.)

Summary

In this unit you have learned that:

- There are a range of services provided for health care, social care and childcare.
- The services provide for the different needs of different people.
- There is a difference between statutory and independent service provision.
- Informal care has an important role in contributing to service provision.
- There are many different job roles in health, social and childcare and there are many different skills required to carry out these roles.
- A progression route is the journey taken to get the qualifications and skills needed to do a particular job role.

Chapter 2

Intro MU 1.2 Understand the principles and values in health and social care (adults and children and young people), early years and childcare

What you will learn in this unit

- The principles and values that support work in health and social care, early years and childcare.
- The guidance and standards that support work in health and social care, early years and childcare.
- Respecting and valuing service users as individuals.
- Person-centred practice.
- How confidentiality helps show respect for individuals.

Important words

Principles and values – The main beliefs and ideas of an organisation

Guidance and standards – Rules and guidelines that should be followed

Respecting and valuing – To show care and consideration of others' views and opinions

Person-centred practice – Listening to a person and meeting their individual needs in the way that is best for them

Confidentiality – Only sharing information with people who need to know or can offer help

Self-esteem – Feeling good about yourself and having confidence

1.1 The principles and values that support work in health and social care and childcare

We all have different principles and values that we learn from the people around us. This might be school rules we have to follow or the way we are expected to behave at home. For example, some families expect shoes to be taken off at the front door, but other families may not think that this is important and wear shoes or boots around the house. Both of these families have principles and values that are different, but are right for them.

When working in health, social care and childcare, it is important to know that we must follow the values and principles of the setting rather than our own.

There are many important principles and values that health, social care and childcare workers need to understand so that they always work in a professional way. This is important to make sure that all children and adults using services are well cared for.

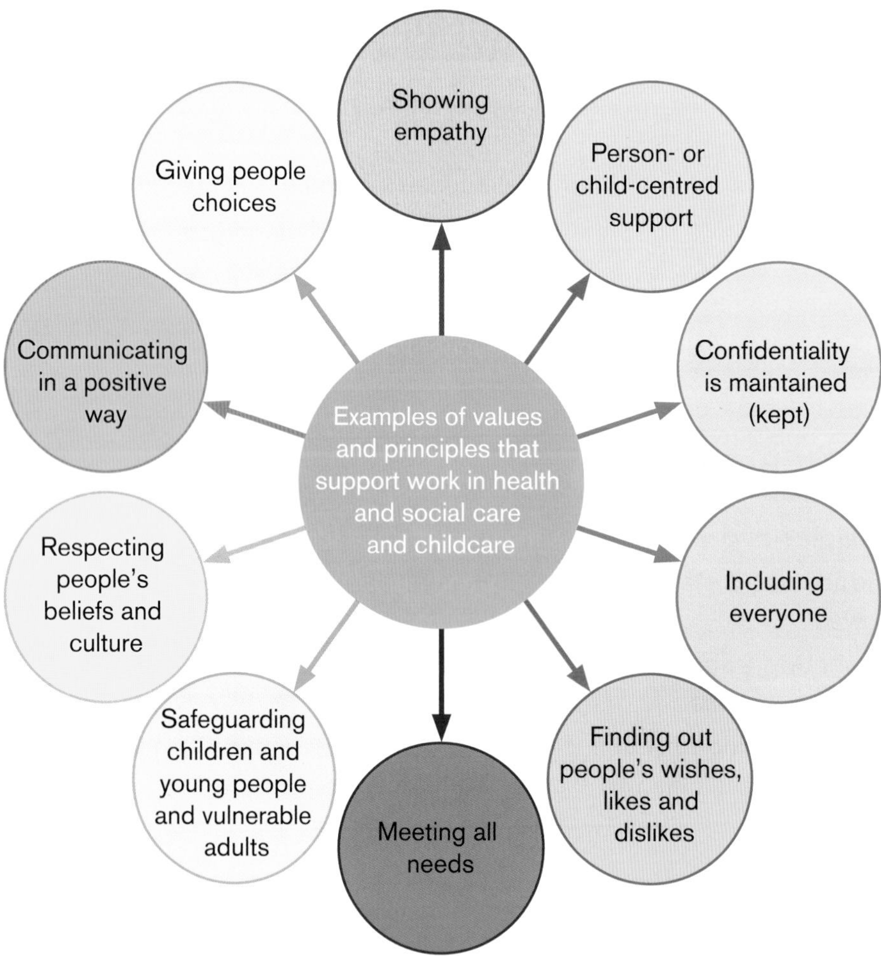

Figure 2.1 Examples of values and principles that support work in health and social care and childcare

1.2 Guidance and standards that support the principles and values

Guidance and standards are the rules that should be understood to make sure that the values and principles are followed by everyone working in the setting.

Equality Act 2010

The Equality Act brings together many different laws linked to equality, diversity and treating people fairly.

This Act is in place to make sure that everyone is treated fairly and is protected from discrimination and includes:

- race
- age
- religion and beliefs
- disablity
- marriage/civil partnership.

Figure 2.2 Equality Act 2010 guidelines

The Early Years Foundation Stage (EYFS)

These are guidelines for good practice which must be followed to meet high standards in childcare.

The EYFS must be followed by most settings caring for and educating children 0–5 years and includes:

- childminders
- day nurseries
- nursery schools.

Figure 2.3 Early Years Foundation Stage guidelines

Health and Social Care Act 2012

This new legislation is about improving the choices and standards of care available.

This Act supports professionals to work in a way that best meets the needs of individuals using the service.

Figure 2.4 Health and Social Care Act standards

Assessment task 1.2 2.1

Make a poster that could be displayed in a staff room in a health centre describing:

- guidance and standards that give us understanding of values and principles in health and social care and childcare
- the values and principles that support work in health and social care and childcare
- why it is important to value and respect service users as individuals.

2.1 Respecting and valuing service users as individuals

The guidance and standards looked at in this chapter are in place to make sure everyone working in health, social care and childcare works in a way that shows respect to, and values the needs and wishes of everyone.

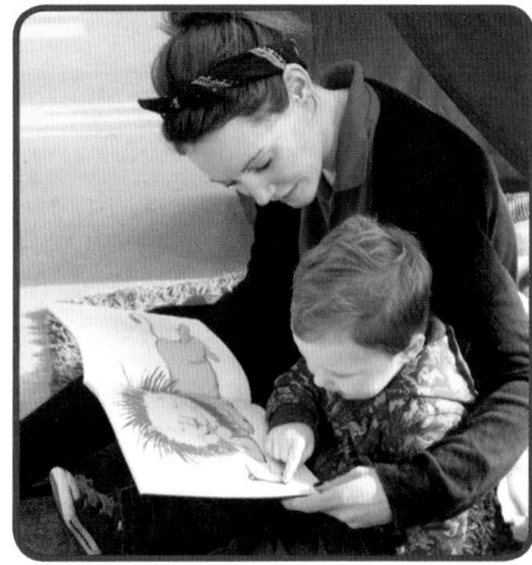

Figure 2.5

It is important that people who use services are respected and valued as individuals so that they **feel valued as people**. By listening to the wishes, needs, likes and dislikes of individuals, and showing you value someone's opinion, that person may **feel more**

confident in making choices for themselves. By showing respect to, and valuing service users, a **more trusting relationship will develop** between them and care workers and this will help the service user to feel more **in control of their own lives.**

When people know that others are interested in their views and opinions, it helps to make them feel respected and valued.

2.2 2.3 Ways to value children, young people and adults

Ways to value children and young people	Ways to value adults
Observe to find out their likes and dislikes	Give them time to speak and listen carefully
Provide activities that they are interested in	Communicate with them in a way that suits their needs
Ask for their opinion and give them choices	Ask about their needs and wishes
Respect cultural and family values	Allow them to make decisions about their daily care routines

Assessment task 2.2 2.3

In pairs, discuss and write down two more ways to:

- value children and young people who access services

Task!

Jack is 77 years old and is moving to an assisted living bungalow. A care worker will help Jack with some of the daily care routines. Give examples of ways that the care worker can show they respect and value Jack.

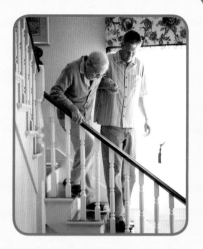

Figure 2.6

2.4 Person-centred practice

Person-centred practice is listening to a person's needs, wishes, likes and dislikes and understanding the importance of meeting their individual needs, in a way that is right for them.

By using **person-centred practice**, the needs and choices of an individual person are seen as very important.

This is very different to not having person-centred practice, where a service may be offered, even if it does not meet all of the person's needs.

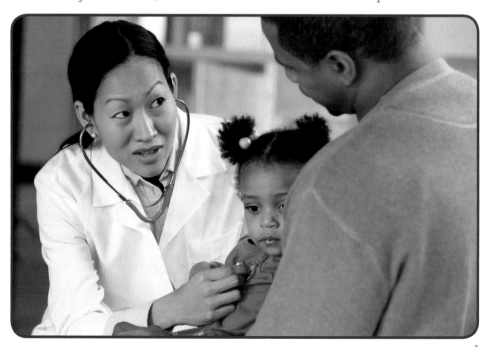

Figure 2.7

Child-centred practice is the same as person-centred practice. This is when the individual care and learning needs of a child are met in a way that is best for them.

An example of child-centred practice is a doctor in a hospital asking a child if they wanted their medicine in a liquid or a tablet, as both are suitable. By allowing the child to make choices about their care, the doctor is valuing their opinion and respecting their wishes.

2.5 Confidentiality

Confidentiality means keeping private information safe and only sharing this information with people who need to know, for example, those who are involved in the health and care of children and adults.

Confidentiality is kept when people working in health, social care and childcare know how to keep information private. All personal information must be stored safely, for example, on a password-protected computer or in a locked cupboard. When you are working in health, social care and childcare you may need to know about a person's family background, health or financial situation, so it is important that you can be always be trusted with personal information.

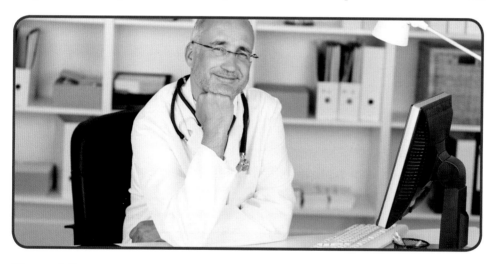

Figure 2.8

2.6 How confidentiality helps show respect for individuals

Confidentiality helps to show respect and values individuals for many reasons; for example, it supports an individual's **self-esteem** because they will feel confident if they know that their private information will only be shared with other professionals who are caring for them.

If an individual thought that their private information was not safe, it could make them feel very worried and affect their confidence and self-esteem.

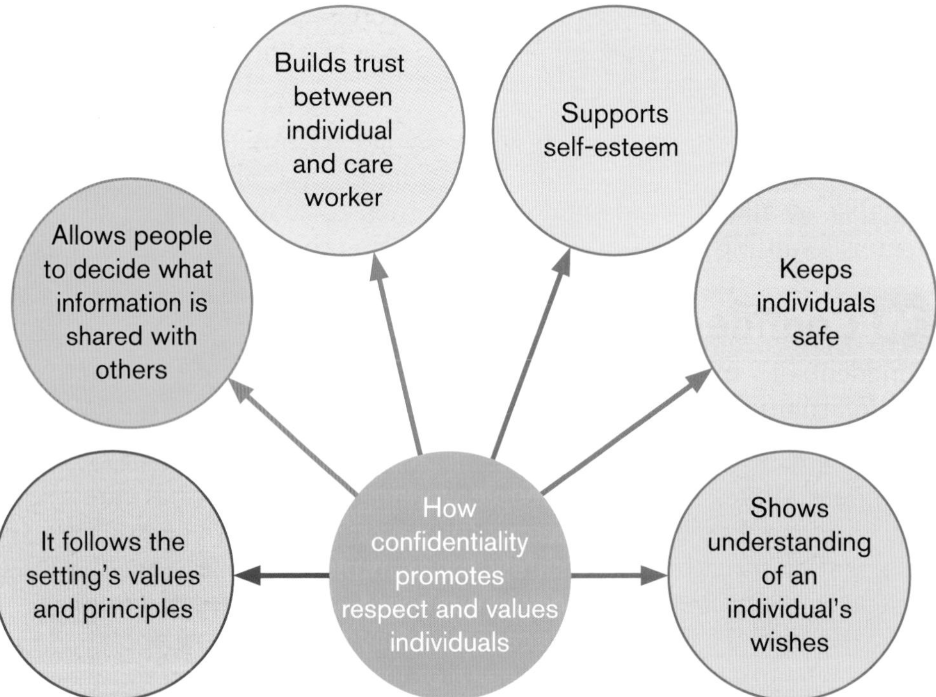

Figure 2.9 How confidentiality promotes respect and values individuals

Assessment task 2.4 2.5 2.6

Create a leaflet for new care workers that includes the following information:

- the meaning of confidentiality in health, social care and childcare
- the meaning of person- and child-centred practice
- describe how confidentiality promotes respect and values individuals.

Summary

In this unit you have learned that:

- There are principles and values that support work in health and social care, early years and childcare.
- The guidance and standards that support work in health and social care, early years and childcare must be followed.
- Respecting and valuing service users as individuals is very important.
- Person-centred practice is about putting the person's needs before the service.
- Confidentiality must be kept to make sure individuals are respected and valued.

Chapter 3

Intro MU 1.4 Awareness of protection and safeguarding in health and social care

What you will learn in this unit

- Keeping children, young people and adults safe from harm, abuse and neglect.
- Signs of harm, abuse and neglect to look out for.
- What to do if you are worried that someone is being harmed, abused or neglected.
- Places that can offer help and information about keeping people safe.

Important words

Harm – Injury or hurt caused to someone

Abuse – To be treated in a damaging way by one or more people

Neglect – This happens when someone is not looked after or cared for properly

Vulnerable person – Someone who could easily be hurt through attack, neglect or unkindness

Safeguarding – Protecting children and adults from harm, abuse or neglect

Support organisations – Organisations such as Childline, NSPCC, Women's Aid which work to protect children and adults

Prevent – Try to stop something from happening

1.1 Protection of vulnerable adults

Protecting vulnerable adults means preventing abuse from taking place or acting quickly when abuse is suspected.

Protecting vulnerable adults is very important when working in health and social care; this is because many people who need health and social care services could easily be hurt or feel hurt by the way they are treated. People using health and social care services often rely on health workers to give them the support they need to be happy and healthy.

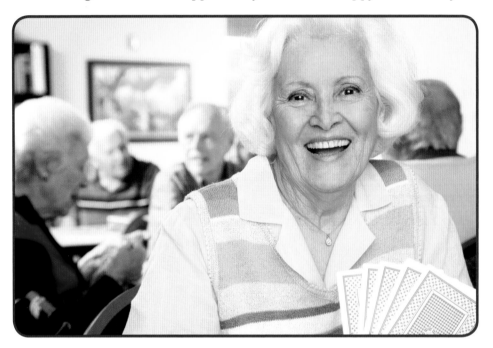

Figure 3.1

Assessment task 1.1 1.2

Produce an information leaflet for health and social care students going into placement for the first time, you need to include a sentence to describe each of these:

- protection of vulnerable adults
- safeguarding children.

1.2 1.3 Safeguarding children and adults from harm, abuse and neglect

Children need protecting from harm, abuse and neglect as they are vulnerable; this is because they are young and are not always able to make choices or decisions for themselves. Protecting children from all types of harm, abuse and neglect is known as **safeguarding**. Responsible and caring adults can help to make sure that the environment and the people in that environment keep children safe.

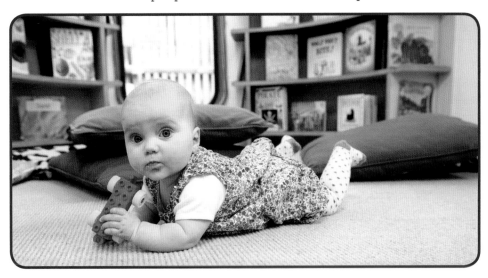

Figure 3.2 Child playing in a safe environment

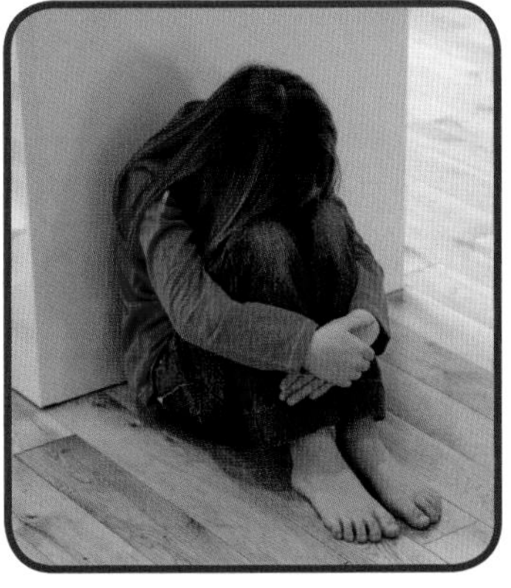

Figure 3.3

Figure 3.4 Power cords should be kept out of reach of children

Harm is when someone gets hurt because of neglect or abuse.

Abuse is when a person or people treat someone very badly. An example of **physical abuse** is when an adult hurts a child on purpose or an older aged adult in a care home is handled roughly. Abuse can also be **emotional abuse**; an example of this is when a person says hurtful words that make someone feel upset or bad about themselves. **Sexual abuse** is when children, young people or vulnerable adults are used for sexual acts or are forced to be involved in making or seeing sexual images.

Neglect is when a person's needs are not met; these may be emotional needs or physical care needs. Children who are neglected will often have health problems such as illness which is not treated or development problems such as not becoming fully toilet trained at the expected age. Adults who are neglected may also become ill due to not being given healthy food or not having enough warmth. Older aged adults may feel neglected or lonely if no one comes to visit them and ignores their needs, such as not getting the help they need to eat, drink, take their medicines or keep themselves clean.

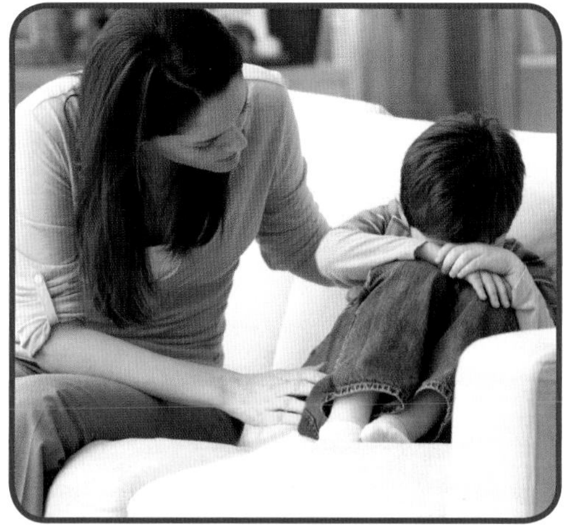

Figure 3.5

Assessment task 1.3

Add information to the leaflet for health and social care students to explain what is meant by 'harm, abuse and neglect' when trying to:

- protect vulnerable adults
- safeguard children.

1.4 Examples of indicators of abuse and neglect

Physical abuse	Emotional abuse	Sexual abuse	Neglect
• Broken bones • Burns, bruises, or bites, which are not explained • Fear • Depression • Untreated injuries • Not wanting to change for PE or swimming lessons	• Depression • Mood changes • Aggressive behaviour • Child becomes clingy • Attention-seeking • Low self-esteem • Sleep or speech problems • Running away • Drug or alcohol misuse	• A child has too much knowledge about sex • Urine infections • Eating problems (anorexia or bulimia) • Sleep problems or nightmares • Bed wetting • Pregnancy • Sexually transmitted diseases	• Hunger/thirst • Poor diet (given only junk food) • Untreated illness • Not being given prescribed medicines • Bed sores • Unwashed clothes • Missing school • Being left alone • Being harmed through unsafe environment

Assessment task 1.4

On the leaflet for health and social care students write down three signs of:

- physical abuse
- emotional abuse
- sexual abuse
- neglect.

Task!

Jamila is being cared for in a residential home. The carers have the job of making sure that the residents are safe and well cared for. Sadly Jamila trips over a wire that is trailing from a heater and burns her leg. Discuss whether you feel this is neglect or an accident.

Ethan, aged two, goes to a local nursery two days each week. His mum collects him in the afternoon and finds that his nappy has not been changed all day. The nappy is heavy and wet and Ethan has a sore nappy rash. Discuss whether you feel this is abuse or neglect or neither.

1.5 Actions to take when there are concerns of harm, abuse or neglect

When someone is worried that a child or adult is at risk of harm, abuse or neglect, there are important steps to take to help that person. It is important to act confidentially: that means that the concerns are not talked about to anyone apart from the setting supervisor, police or professionals from support organisations.

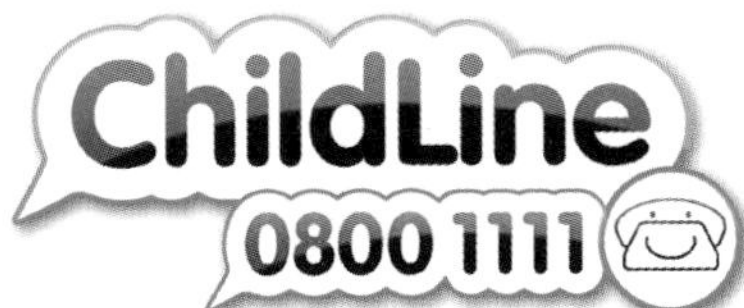
ChildLine
0800 1111

Figure 3.6

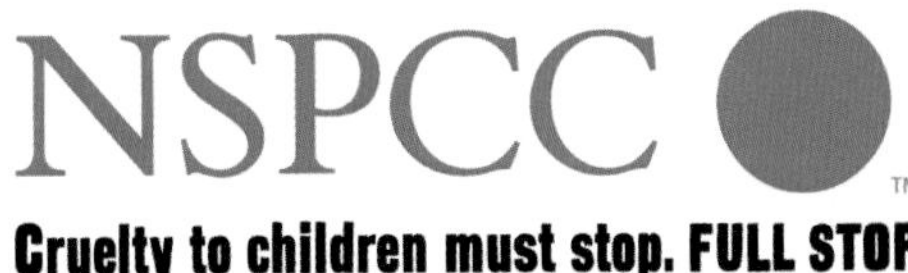
NSPCC
Cruelty to children must stop. FULL STOP.

Figure 3.7

When there is a concern about a person being harmed, abused or neglected, the first step is to write down the facts. If the concern is in the work place, for example, in a children's nursery, a hospital or a residential home, the first action would be to talk to the supervisor or the person responsible for safeguarding, clearly explaining what the concerns are. The person responsible for dealing with reports of abuse or neglect will investigate the concern and tell the police, social services or other organisations, if necessary.

If the concern relates to something outside of work, it is still important to report it. The police force has officers who are experienced in dealing with protection and safeguarding of adults and children. There are many organisations such as Childline, NSPCC, Refuge and Women's Aid which offer online advice and telephone helplines to use when there are concerns about a person's safety. Again, it is important that the concerns are not discussed with anyone other than the people who can help, as confidentiality must be kept.

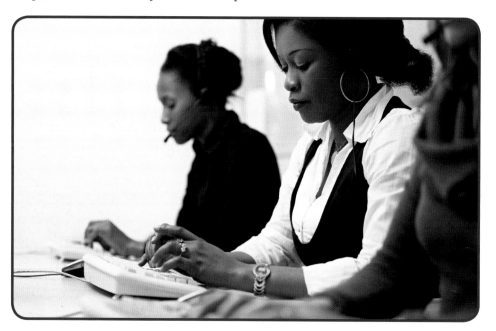

Figure 3.8 Telephone helplines

Assessment task 1.5

On the leaflet for health and social care students write down what the students should do if they are worried about someone being harmed, abused or neglected.

1.6 Confidentiality

Confidentiality means only sharing information with people who need to know or can offer help and support. The person responsible for protection and safeguarding in the workplace will have a very good understanding of confidentiality and will know what to do to keep information private. If someone is at risk of serious harm or abuse, the information will be shared quickly with the police or other organisations that can help to keep the person safe or get them to a safe place quickly. All personal information must be stored safely, for example, on a password-protected computer or in a locked cupboard.

Assessment task 1.6

On the leaflet for health and social care students write down:

- why it is important to understand confidentiality
- when it is important to share information.

1.7 Responsibility for safeguarding

Information should only be shared with people who need to know the facts or who can offer protection, such as the police, child protection officers, social services, safeguarding professionals or setting managers. Sometimes the setting managers, social services or the police will decide to share the information with parents or main carers if they think it is necessary.

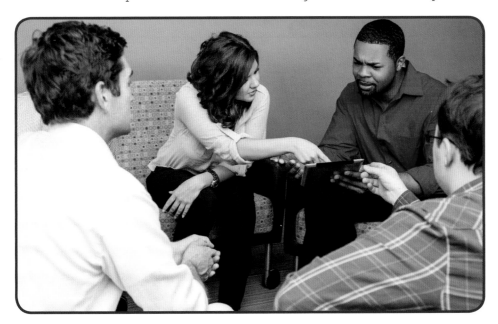

Figure 3.9

Task!

In pairs or small groups, read the information above and make a list of people or organisations responsible for protecting vulnerable adults and safeguarding children.

Assessment task 1.7

On the leaflet you are making include some information about the people who have responsibility for safeguarding.

1.8 The role of organisations in safeguarding

Organisations such as schools, nurseries, care homes, day care centres for older aged adults and adults with disabilities all have a responsibility to protect children and adults. To protect everyone, organisations should have written policies which describe how to protect and safeguard everyone working in or using the service. Each setting will have written guidance which clearly explains what should be done when there is a concern about harm, abuse or neglect. Everyone who works in any of these organisations or settings will have safeguarding training so everyone knows what to do if they have a concern. This guidance or training will also include steps to take if someone is worried that a care worker is not treating people properly, for example, shouting unkindly at a child or not taking care of a vulnerable adult.

Task!

A care worker goes into the home of an older aged man most days to help him to get showered and dressed. The care worker is worried when the man tells her that he is glad that she has come today, because the other care worker shouts at him for being too slow and that she sometimes hurts him when she helps him dress.

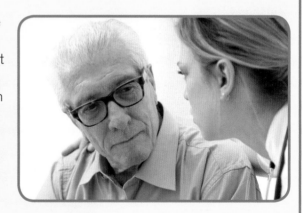

Figure 3.10

What should the care worker do now that she knows this might be happening?

Assessment task 1.8

On the leaflet for health and social care students write down:

- what organisations can do to protect children and vulnerable adults.

1.9 Support available for people experiencing harm, abuse or neglect

Support is also available for people who deal with cases of harm, abuse or neglect as they too may be affected in some way; for example, they may feel upset or concerned that they should have been able to do more to help.

Examples of sources of support include:

Information

The Samaritans

The Samaritans are a charity available 24 hours a day offering confidential advice and support to anyone in distress. They also work to raise awareness of issues such as suicide and depression.
www.samaritans.org

Seeking counselling?

Your GP

Remember that your own GP or health centre are good places to find out what NHS-funded services you may be able to access with a GP referral.

Worried about a young person being bullied or abused?

Kidscape

Kidscape is committed to keeping children safe from abuse. Kidscape is the first charity in the UK established specifically to prevent bullying and child sexual abuse. The helpline is for the use of parents, guardians or concerned relatives and friends of bullied children. If you are a child and are experiencing bullying problems, then please visit or ring Childline.

Worried about a young person?

ChildLine

Whatever your worry, it's better out than in. Call ChildLine for help.
www.childline.org.uk

NSPCC

The aim of the National Society for the Prevention of Cruelty to Children (NSPCC) is to protect children from cruelty, support vulnerable families, campaign for changes to the law and raise awareness about abuse.
www.nspcc.org.uk

Worried about a vulnerable adult?

Voice UK

A national charity that supports people with learning disabilities and other vulnerable people who have experienced crime or abuse. It also supports their families, carers and professional workers.
www.voiceuk.org.uk

Source: Information from www.excellencegateway.org.uk

Task!

Can you find out about other sources of support or information about protection and safeguarding?

You could look for leaflets in doctors' surgeries, Citizens Advice centres or chemists, or search for information on the internet.

Assessment task 1.9

At the end of your leaflet list some sources of support linked to protection and safeguarding.

Summary

In this unit you have learned that:

- It is important to keep children, young people and vulnerable adults safe from harm, abuse and neglect.
- There are many ways that harm, abuse and neglect can take place and there are many signs that show this may be happening.
- It is important to take the right actions if you are worried that someone is being harmed, abused or neglected.
- Confidentiality is very important and information must be shared and stored safely.
- There are many professions and organisations that offer support and help to keep people safe.

Chapter 4

Intro MU 1.6 Introduction to communication in health and social care (adults and children and young people), early years and childcare

What you will learn in this unit

- Different ways to communicate with children and adults.
- Barriers that stop communication happening.
- Methods that may help to break down communication barriers.

Important words

Verbal communication – Speaking and listening

Non-verbal communication – Ways to communicate without speaking

Informal communication – Speaking with friends

Formal communication – this is when information is shared in a professional way. Slang words are not used

Communication methods – Ways to communicate

What is communication? Communication is a way of getting or giving information.

Good communication is very important when you are working with others or looking after people. You often need to get information from people such as what they want to do, or how they feel. You might need to give information to others, for example, telling them the time of their appointment or where the bus will pick them up.

1.1 Communication methods

People communicate with each other in lots of different ways and for lots of different reasons. These methods may include:

Verbal communication – This is when information is given thorough speaking and listening.

Non-verbal communication – This is when information is given through body language, hand gestures and facial expressions.

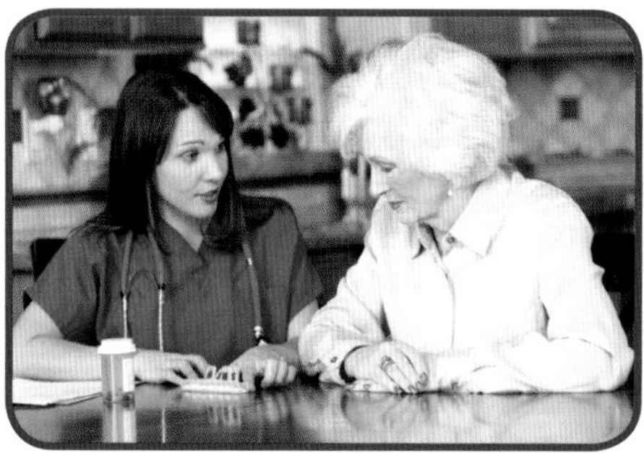

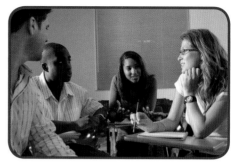

Figure 4.1 The nurse is asking this person how she feels

Figure 4.2 The health care students are sharing their ideas

Task!

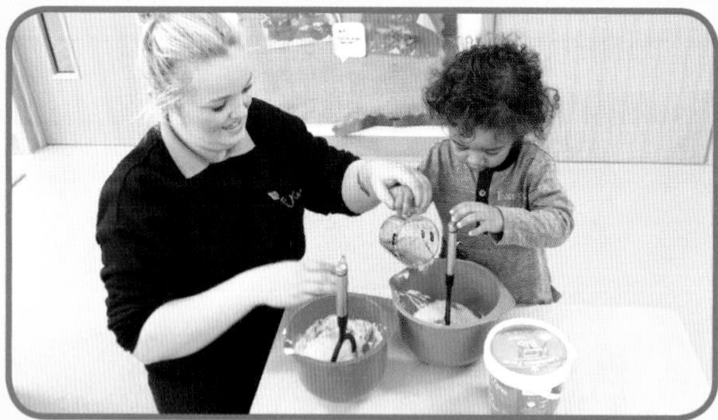

Figure 4.3

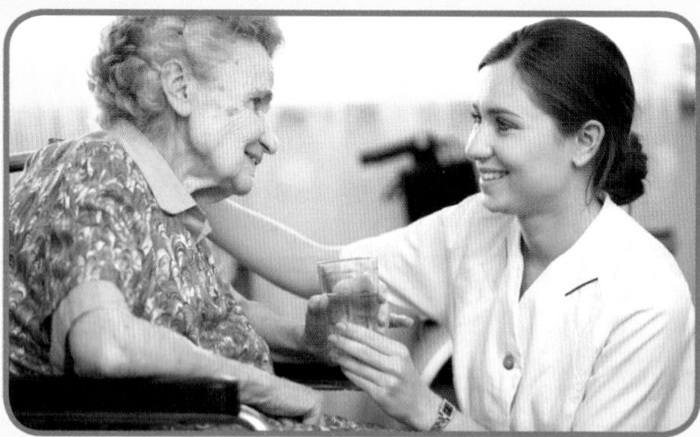

Figure 4.3

Can you decide what the people are trying to say through their body language and hand gestures?

Sometimes other types of non-verbal communication are needed; for example, a hearing-impaired person may use sign language such as Makaton to communicate.

Written communication – This is when information is written down. This can be handwritten, for example, a shopping list, or printed, perhaps from a computer or in a newspaper.

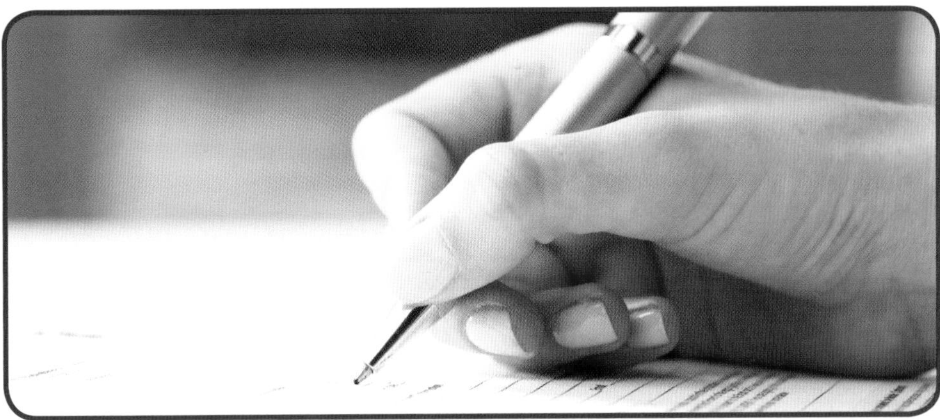

Figure 4.5 Handwritten information

Pictures and visual communication – This is when information is given through pictures and signs.

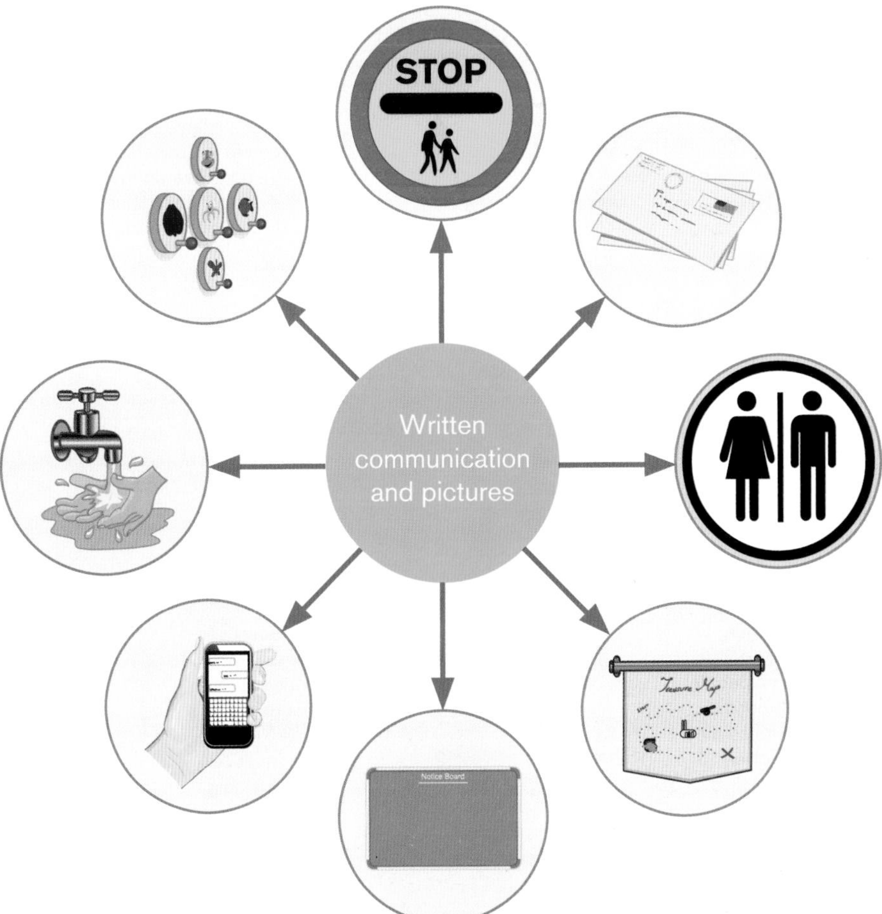

Figure 4.6 Written communication and pictures

Task!

Can you think of any other examples of communication using pictures or signs?

Assessment task 1.1

Make a spider diagram identifying at least five different communication methods.

Skills needed to communicate

There are lots of skills needed to communicate well. These include those listed in the figure below.

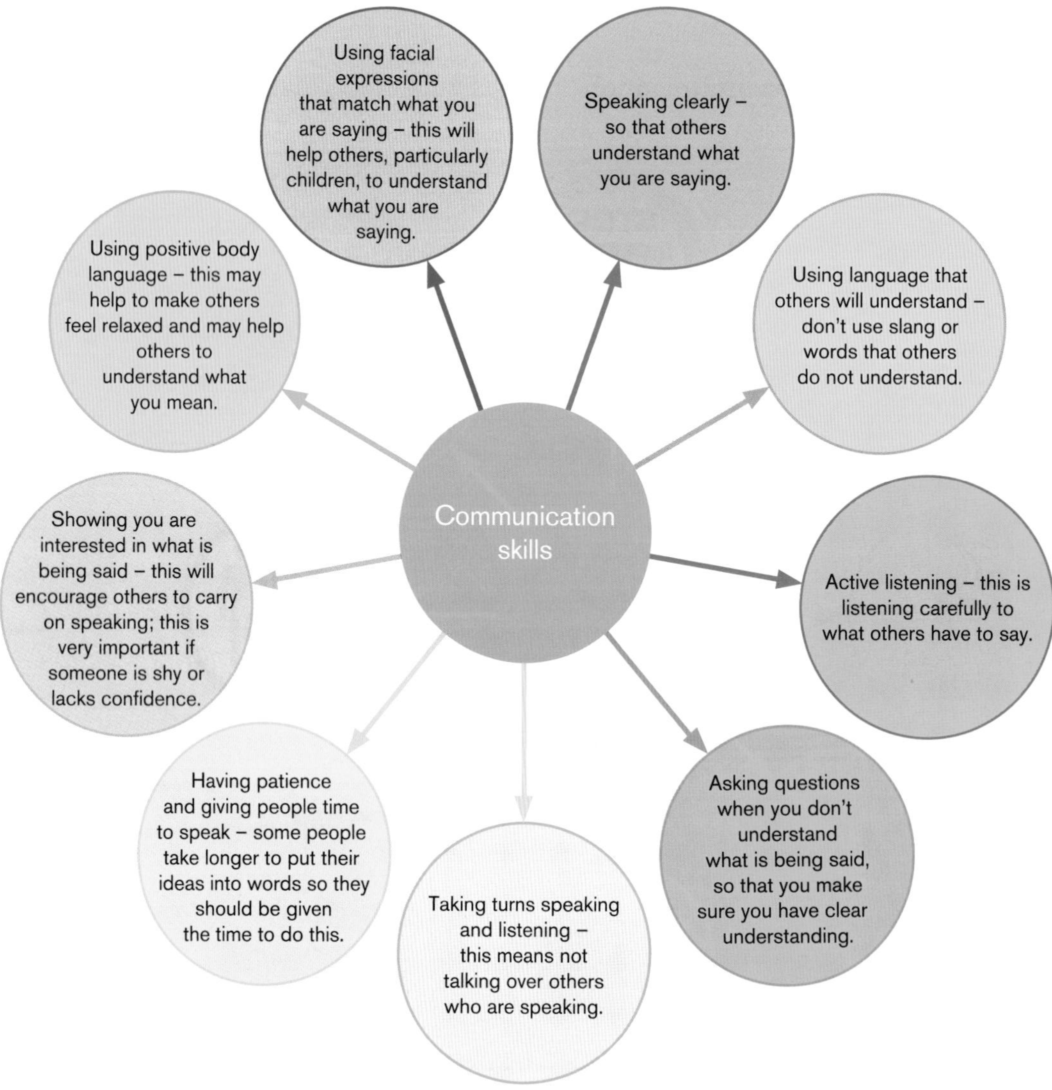

Figure 4.7 Communication skills

Types of communication include:

One to one: This means two people are having a conversation. To do this well, each person will be talking clearly, listening carefully, using facial expressions (for example, smiling) and using body language (for example, nodding your head, or using hand movements).

Group discussions: This is when communication is taking place with more than one person, for example, a teacher explaining the rules of a game to a group of children, or a team of carers discussing how to improve the menus for the older aged residents in the care home.

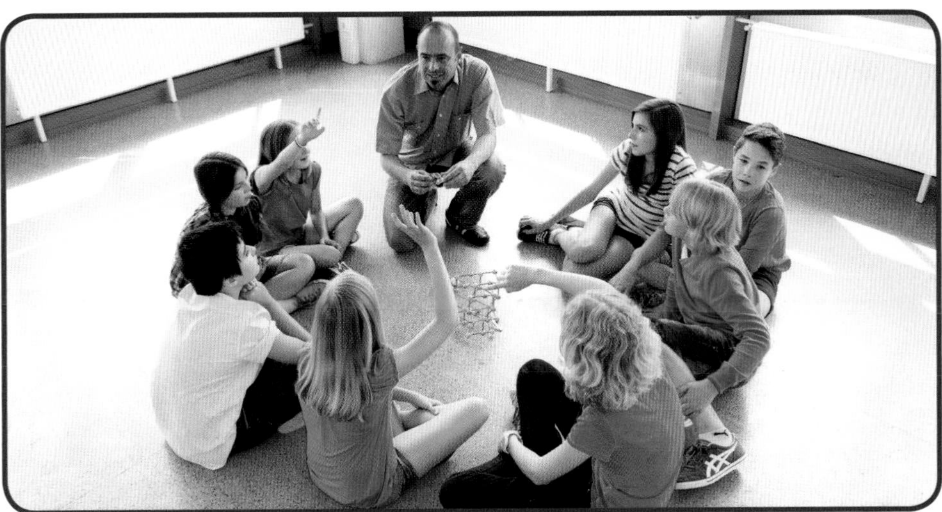

Figure 4.8 The teacher is using clear language that the children can understand

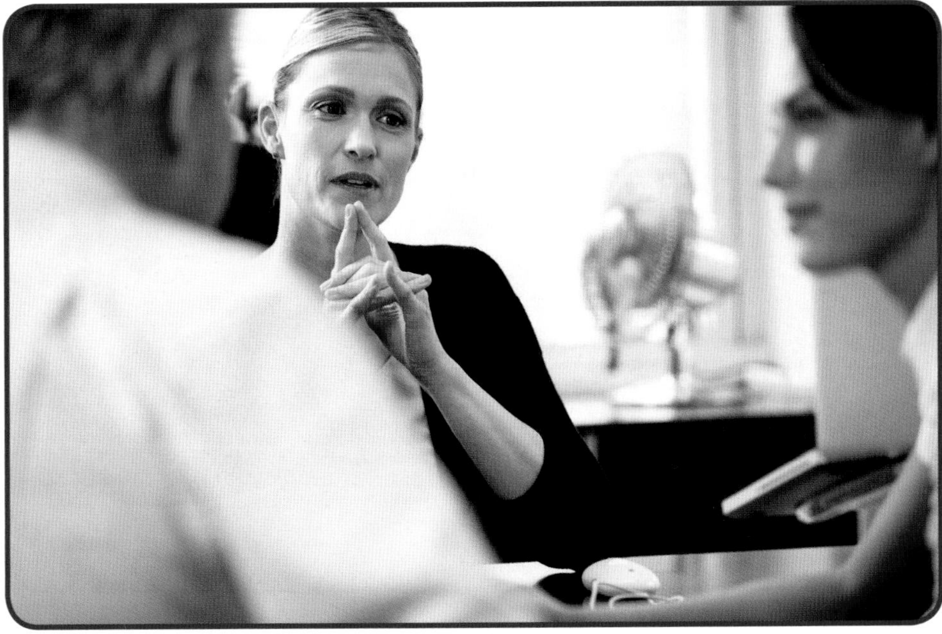

Figure 4.9 The manager is listening to everyone's ideas

Informal communication

This usually takes place between people who know each other well or between family members, for example, friends chatting in the park or a family talking during meal times.

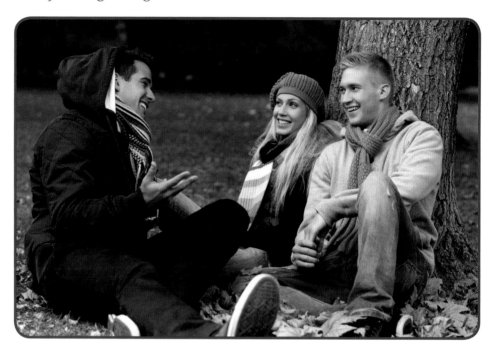

Figure 4.10 Friends chatting in the park

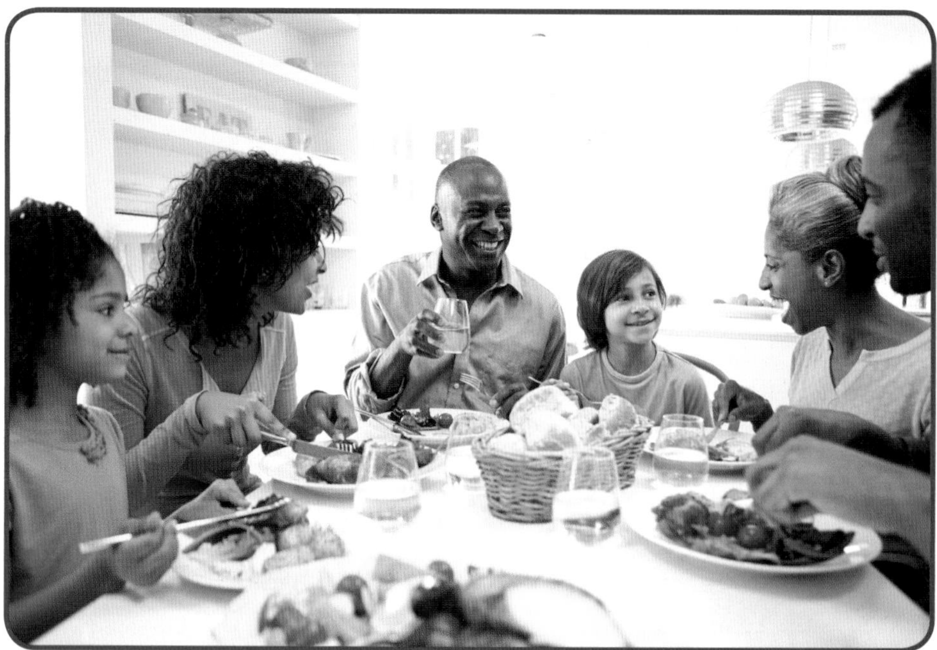

Figure 4.11 Family talking during meal time

Formal communication

Formal communication often happens in the workplace, for example, a midwife in a health centre discussing care needs with a pregnant woman. Another example of formal communication is when a group of early years workers meet with the nursery manager to plan play activities for children. During formal communication it is important to speak clearly and to use appropriate language. This is because communication is an important part of being a care professional.

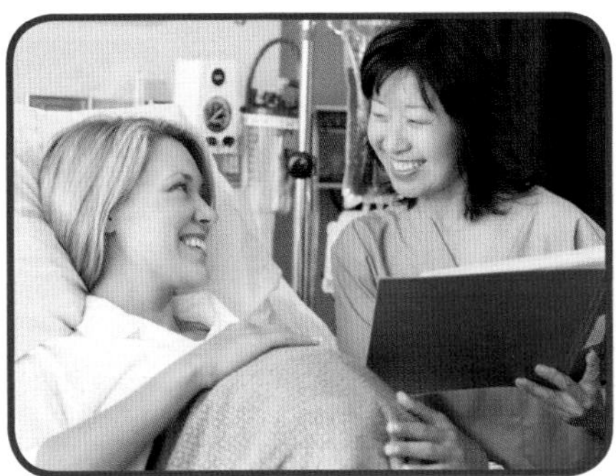

Figure 4.12 The midwife needs to give the pregnant woman information about a healthy diet

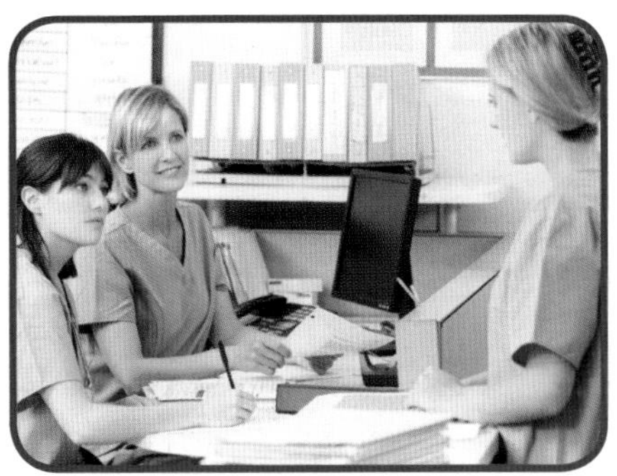

Figure 4.13 The nursery manager asks the team to share their ideas

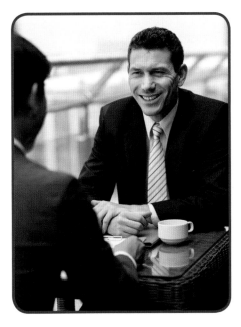

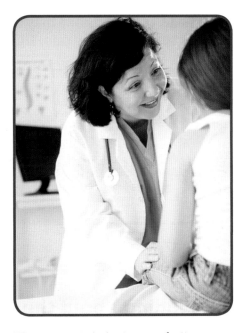

Figure 4.14 Two friends meeting for coffee

Figure 4.15 A doctor comforting a patient

Figure 4.16 A childminder and a child, playing

When people communicate in groups, it is important that everyone is given the chance to speak and be listened to. This is a good way for lots of ideas or feelings to be shared, especially when important decisions need to be made. Often someone may be very good at speaking but not good at listening to what is being said. This is a barrier to communication.

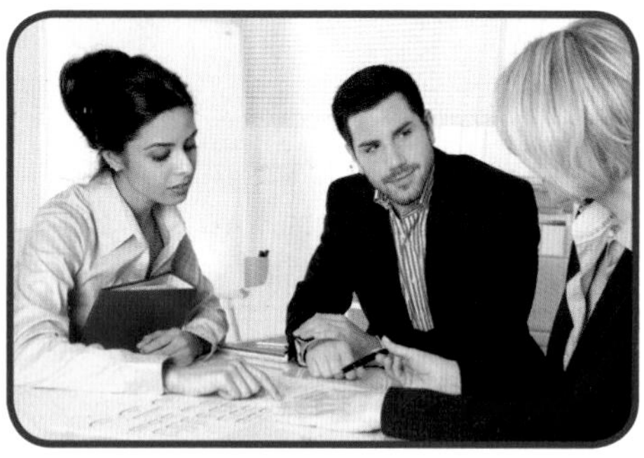

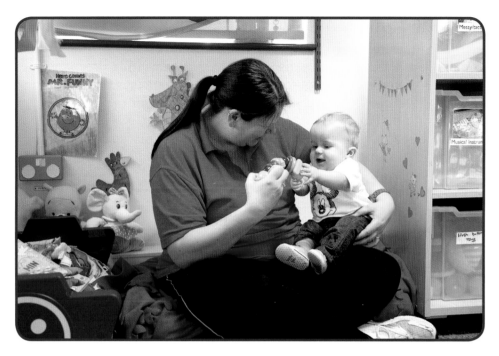

Figure 4.17 Social workers discussing the needs of families

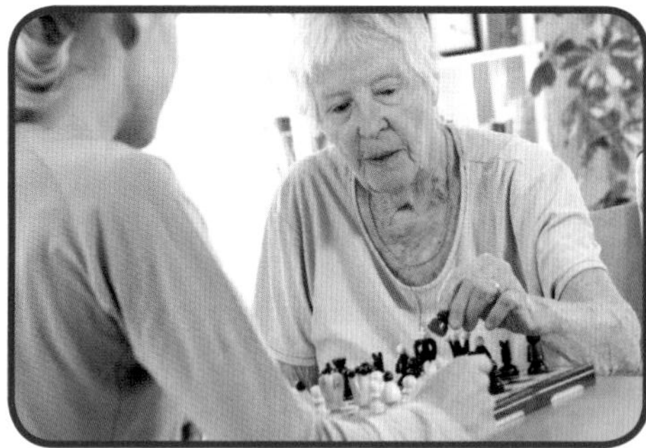

Figure 4.18 A carer supporting an activity

2.1 Finding about the communication needs of individuals

Communication is very important in health and social care and early years care. By taking time to find out about how best to communicate with someone, or finding ways to help a person communicate and be understood, you may make life a lot happier for someone who usually finds communication difficult.

It is very important to find out the communication and language needs of others. This could include understanding ways to improve communication with a person.

Ways to improve communication	Example
Ask questions	What time would you like your lunch?
Observe the individual	Watch the child communicate with friends to see how their language skills are developing
Ask other people who may have useful information	Ask parents or family members how best to communicate with a person close to them
Talk to the carers of individuals	
Read case notes or personal records	

Table 4.1 Understanding ways to improve communication with a person

Just by asking questions about how best to communicate with someone will help to support good communication. Sometimes others such as parents, family or support services can help you to understand how best to communicate with someone. Health care workers will often look at a person's records or care plan to see if there is any information about how best to communicate with that person.

Identifying individual communication needs

When working with people of all ages, from babies to older aged adults or people with disabilities, it is really important to communicate in an appropriate way so that good communication takes place. It is important to use good communication skills so that the correct information is given and easily understood. Some people have different communication needs and it is the job of a health care or early years worker to find out these needs and look for ways to communicate well.

Parents and carers use a type of communication with babies called 'parentese'. This involves speaking in a higher than usual pitch, sometimes in a sing-song voice, often repeating words or simple sentences.

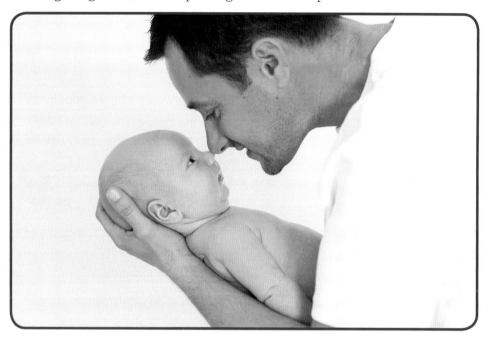

Figure 4.19 Parents use a type of communication called 'parentese'

The parents or carer will give lots of eye contact and use lots of positive facial expressions such as smiling. Babies communicate through different sounding cries, and as they begin to gurgle and babble, this is the beginning of communication skills.

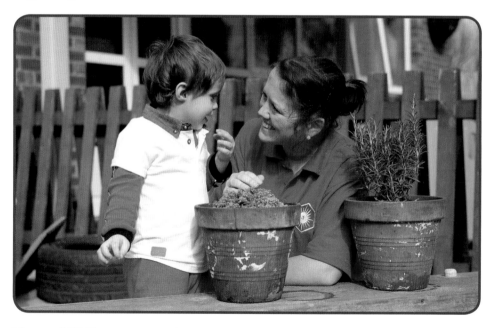

Figure 4.20 Eye contact and smiling are important

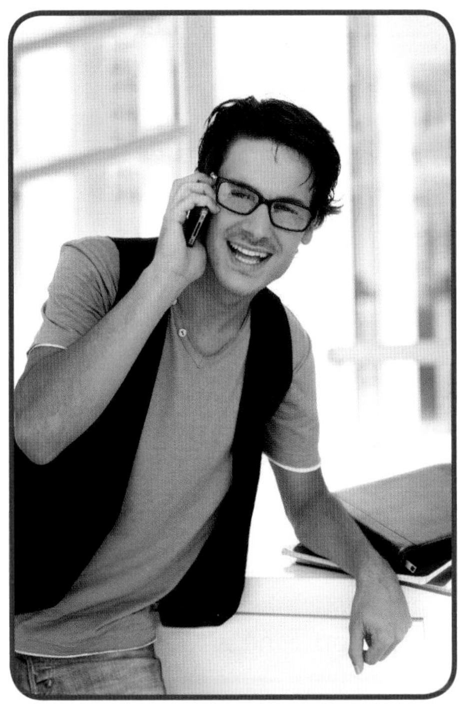

Figure 4.21 Young people often use mobile phones to text or talk

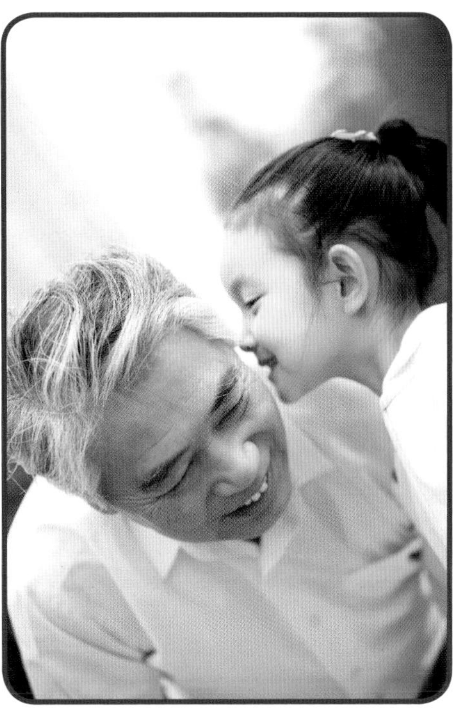

Figure 4.22 Hearing impairments can make communication difficult

Some young people prefer to communicate with their friends through the use of mobile phones to text or talk, or through a computer to email or access social media websites.

Communication impairments

When a person has a hearing impairment, they may find communication difficult. Often a person will use some type of hearing aid to help them hear more easily. Sign language such as Makaton can be used to help children with communication difficulties.

Some children's TV programmes support children with communication needs by using Makaton. See **www.bbc.co.uk/cbeebies/something-special/**

Assessment task 2.1

Robin is 14 years old. He has hearing and speech impairment and finds communicating difficult. Robin cannot always easily communicate his needs, wishes and preferences.

How could you identify Robin's communication and language needs, wishes and preferences?

2.2 2.3 Barriers to communication and overcoming barriers to communication

A barrier to communication is anything that stops good communication taking place.

This could be a language barrier, where perhaps two people speak different languages; an environmental barrier such as a very noisy room; or an emotional barrier when perhaps someone is too upset to give or receive communication.

Another barrier could be a physical barrier when perhaps someone is visually impaired and cannot see the facial expressions or body language which would make it difficult to understand if someone was being serious or not. A hearing barrier is when a person is not able to hear clearly, or perhaps has no hearing at all.

A cultural barrier is when an acceptable way to communicate in some cultures, such as pointing to a sign, is seen as rude by other cultures. In most cultures it is important to give good eye contact when speaking; however, in a few cultures giving eye contact to other people when speaking is seen as very rude.

Social barriers could include using words that others do not understand or speaking in a way that makes others feel uncomfortable.

It is important to find ways to overcome barriers to communication so that a person's needs, wishes and preferences can be identified.

Barriers to communication	**Ways to overcome the barriers to communication**
Children, older adults or wheelchair users who may be lower down than others	Make sure you get down to the same level as others so that you can make good eye contact and allow the child or person to feel included
	Use an interpreter to communicate information
Loud, noisy room where it is difficult to clearly hear what others are saying	
Cultural differences in using hand signs or eye contact	Be aware that some cultures have different meanings for some hand signs and that eye contact can be seen as threatening or disrespectful within some cultures
Not showing respect	Make sure you ask a person the name they prefer you to use when speaking to them, e.g. Mrs Green rather than saying 'Sunita' or 'love'
Chairs placed too far apart or not facing each other	
When people use slang words or complicated words	
	Make sure that if the person uses a hearing aid, it is switched on Use sign language or other communication methods that the person prefers
Lack of confidence in communicating with other people, for example, speaking in a group or talking to a doctor or social worker	Using positive facial expressions, such as smiling, and positive body language, such as nodding, may help a person feel more relaxed

Table 4.2 Barriers to communication and how they can be overcome

Assessment task 2.2 2.3

Complete the table above to show barriers to communication and ways to overcome these barriers.

Summary

In this unit you have learned that:

- There are many different ways to communicate with children and adults.
- People may have individual communication and language needs and preferences that should be recognised.
- There are a range of barriers that stop effective communication.
- Barriers to communication can be overcome when appropriate ways to communicate are found.

Chapter 5

PWCS 03 Introductory awareness of equality and inclusion in health, social care and children's and young people's settings

What you will learn in this unit

- The importance of equality and inclusion within health, social care and children's and young people's settings.
- The effects of discriminatory attitudes and behaviours on individuals.
- Social and physical barriers that may prevent equality and inclusion.
- Ways to overcome barriers that prevent equality and inclusion.
- The behaviours that may promote equality and inclusion.

Important words

Equality – Making sure all people are treated fairly

Inclusion – Making sure everyone can be included

Discriminatory attitudes and behaviour – When someone judges another person or group of people because of the way they look, how they speak, the music they listen to or the clothes they choose to wear

Legislation – Laws or rules which must be followed

Principles and values – The main beliefs and ideas of an organisation

Barrier – Something that gets in a person's way and may stop them from doing something

Social barrier – The way people are treated by others which can stop them being included or taking part in an activity

Physical barrier – When someone is stopped from taking part in an activity because the environment and/or equipment does not meet their individual needs

1.1 1.2 Equality and inclusion and how they form the basis for the principles and values of health, social care and children's and young people's settings

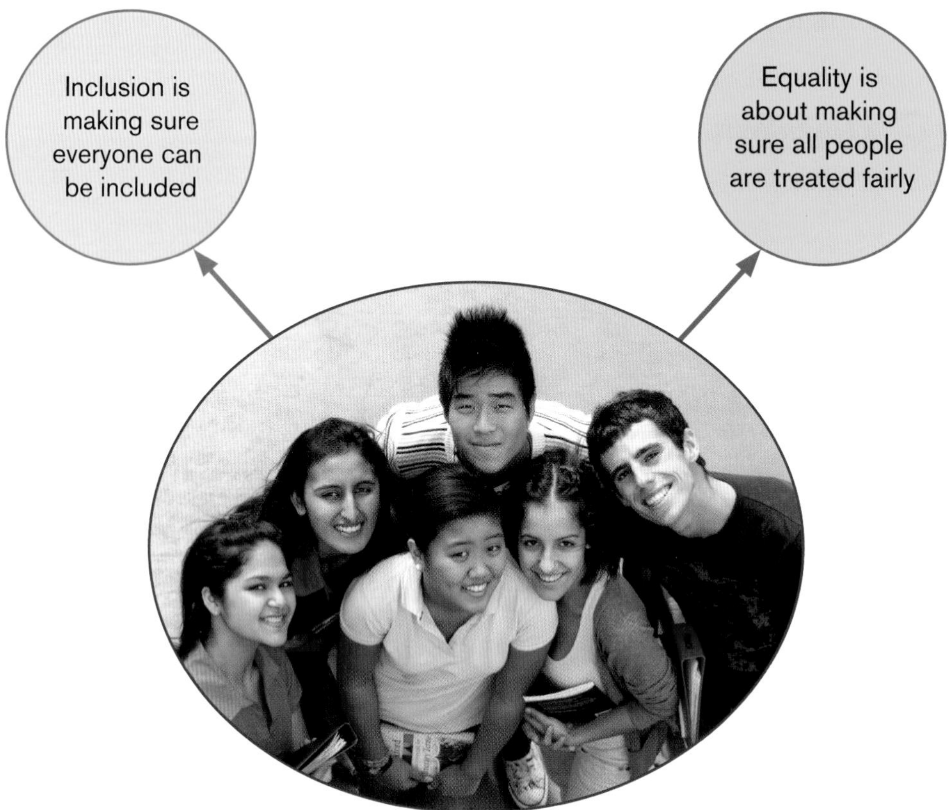
Inclusion is making sure everyone can be included
Equality is about making sure all people are treated fairly

Figure 5.1 Equality and inclusion

All organisations have principles and values, which everyone should be aware of, to help them to work in a way that is both fair and meets the needs of everyone using the service.

To understand that equality and inclusion should be included in the principles and values of a setting, it is first important to know that there is legislation (laws) that has been created to support equality and inclusion. This important legislation MUST be followed and includes:

- Equality Act 2012
- Early Years Foundation Stage 2012
- Health and Social Care Act 2012.

Assessment task 1.1 1.2

Make a colourful poster for the wall which shows:

- the meaning of the terms 'equality' and 'inclusion'
- how equality and inclusion should be included in a setting's values and principles.

2.1 Discriminatory attitudes

Discrimination is the treatment of an individual based on the group or category to which the person belongs. For example:

- age
- gender
- language
- cultural background
- religion
- disability.

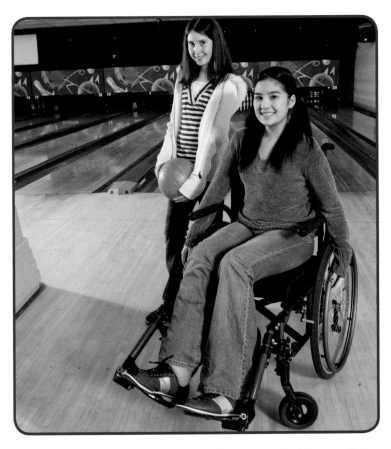

Figure 5.2 A wheelchair bound girl being included in an activity

A discriminatory attitude is when someone judges another person or group of people because of the way they look, how they speak, the music they listen to or the clothes they choose to wear.

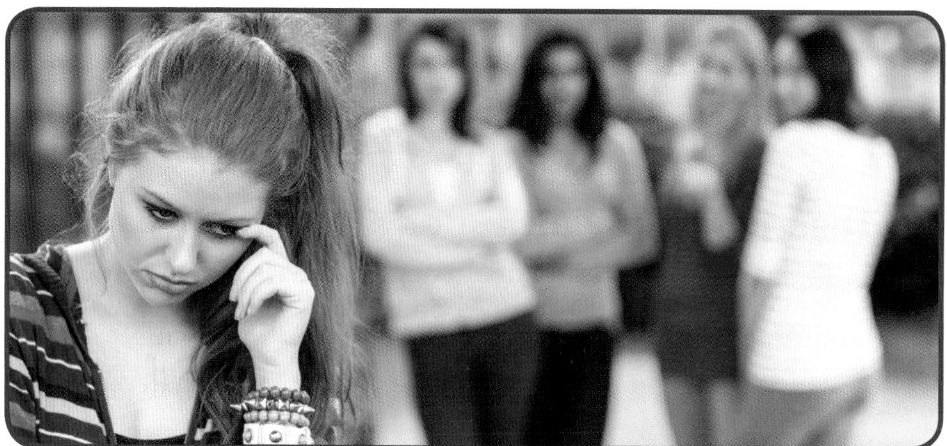

Figure 5.3

2.2 How discriminatory attitudes can affect individuals

When a person is discriminated against, they may feel left out of the group or they may feel no one understands them. This may make them feel very unhappy or very bad about themselves.

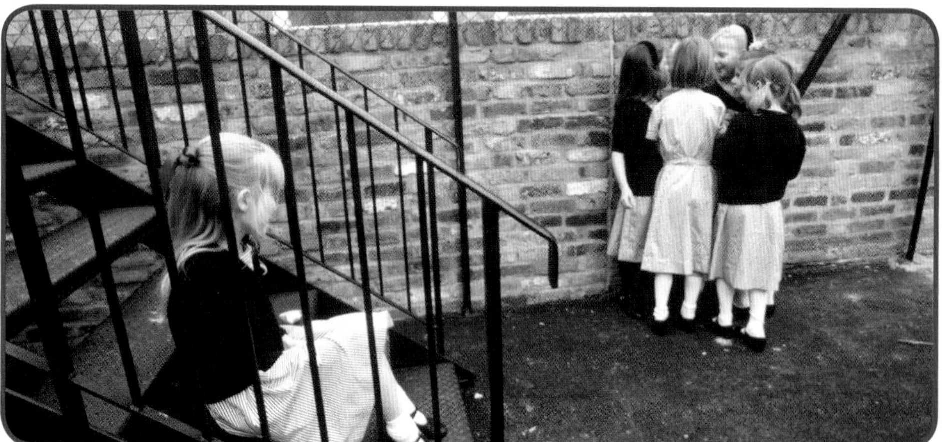

Figure 5.4

Being discriminated against can make a person feel worthless and they may choose not to get involved in activities in the setting or mix with others in the group. This could affect their care or education because they may not feel they want to attend the setting. They may become isolated and want to stay in their own home; they may feel afraid for their safety, or even become ill.

Assessment task 2.1 2.2

Using the information you have read in sections 2.1 and 2.2, complete the table below by identifying how discriminatory attitudes can affect individuals.

Identify discriminatory attitudes	Give examples of how discriminatory attitudes can affect individuals
age	
language	

2.3 Discriminatory behaviours

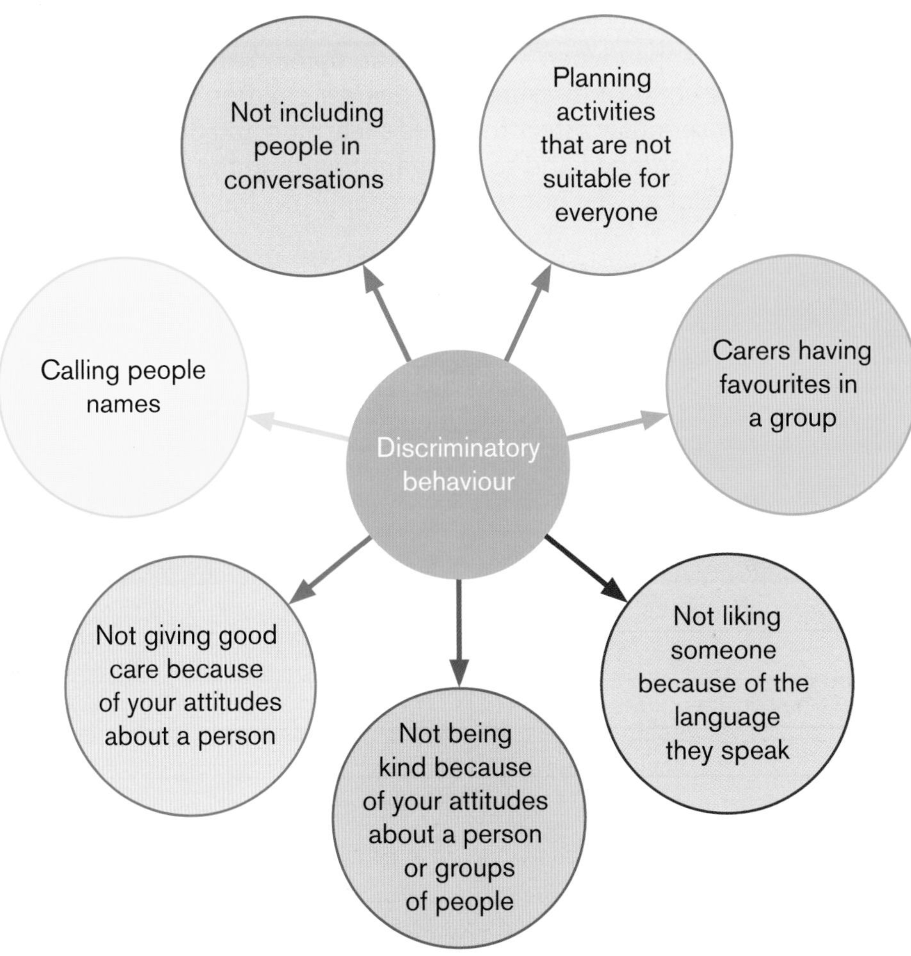

Figure 5.5 Discriminatory behaviours

2.4 How discriminatory behaviours can affect individuals

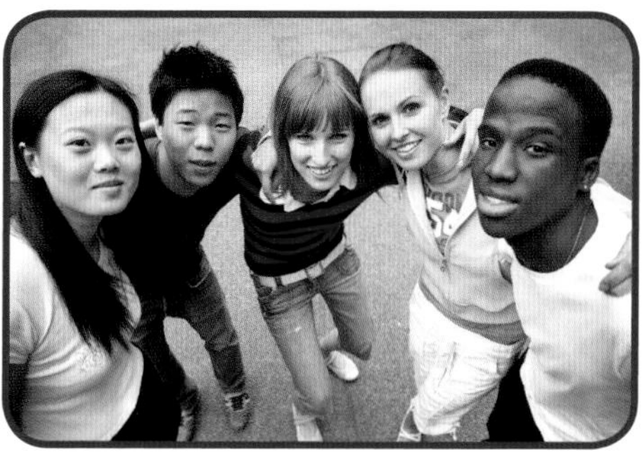

Figure 5.6

Discriminatory behaviours may result in someone not having the care and help that they need and deserve. The person may feel very unhappy or their needs may not be met and they may be neglected or even worse become ill. For example, if a carer does not give the time and care to a person, they may not notice a health problem or may forget to give out medication. This is very poor practice and the carer could damage the individual's health or they could lose their job. Because discrimination is against the law, carers who discriminate could even be taken to court.

Children may also be affected by discriminatory behaviours in the setting. This may happen when a carer has an opinion about the family background of the child, or discriminates against children from a different culture. This may seriously affect the child's learning and development. The child may be frightened and so not want to attend the setting; they may become withdrawn and not trust the people around them.

Assessment task 2.3 2.4

Using the information in sections 2.3 and 2.4, complete the table below to identify how discriminatory attitudes can affect individuals.

Identify discriminatory behaviours	Give examples of how discriminatory behaviours can affect individuals
Calling people names	
Carers having favourites	

3.1 Social and physical barriers that may prevent equality and inclusion

Social barriers that may prevent equality and inclusion in settings can be something as simple as not being made to feel welcome within a group. Social barriers can also include not having the confidence to join in with activities or talk to others in the group.

If a carer or other person in the group has acted in a discriminatory way towards an individual, the individual may feel afraid to join in, or may want to stay out of the way in case something happens to upset them.

Another social barrier might be a learning difficulty, which means that a person is not able to communicate or socialise with others confidently. People with a sight or hearing impairment may not have an equal chance to take part in all activities if their needs are not met when activities or routines are provided.

Physical barriers may include having a physical disability which is not thought about by carers when they are planning activities for the whole group. Other physical barriers include not having the special equipment needed or enough space to move around safely.

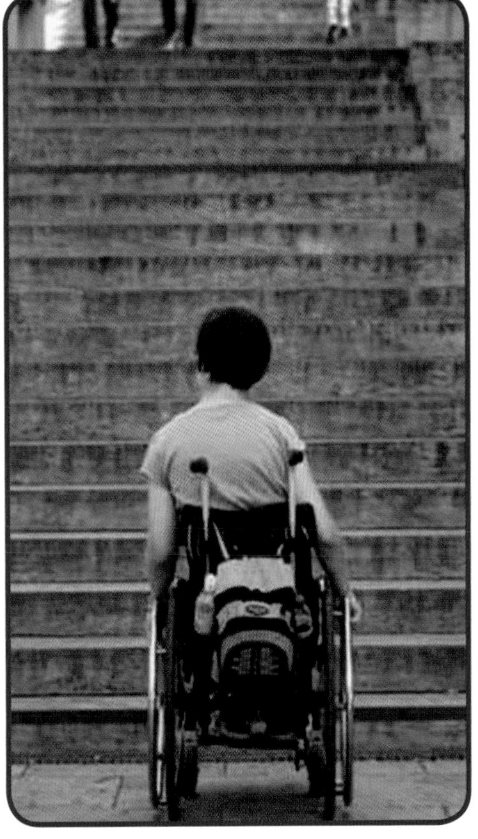

Figure 5.7

3.2 How barriers to equality and inclusion may be overcome

All barriers to equality and inclusion can be overcome by using a person-centred approach when planning activities and providing care. It is important that carers think about the individual needs and skills of every person in the group and find ways to make sure they are all included.

Carers may need to find out about any special equipment that might help a person to feel included. Equality and inclusion training is important for carers to understand how they can find out about the needs of children and young people and meet those needs.

3.3 Behaviours that may promote equality and inclusion

Carers as professionals must be good role models and always include everyone in activities and routines. When carers behave in a positive way and treat everyone fairly, others will see that this is the right way to treat people and will copy this behaviour. Carers must act quickly to stop any discriminatory behaviour.

If carers do not step in when they see discriminatory behaviour, others in the group may think it is acceptable to behave this way and people could carry on being hurt.

Assessment task 3.1 3.2 3.3

Create a leaflet which gives information about equality and inclusion. The leaflet should include:

- social and physical barriers that may prevent equality and inclusion
- how these barriers can be removed
- positive behaviour that supports equality and inclusion.

Summary

In this unit you have learned that:

- It is important to maintain equality and inclusion in health, social care and children's and young people's settings.
- Discriminatory attitudes and behaviour can hurt individuals.
- Social and physical barriers may stop equality and inclusion.
- There are many ways to remove the barriers which prevent equality and inclusion.
- People's behaviour can promote equality and inclusion.

Chapter 6

PWCS 04 Introductory awareness of health and safety in health, social care and children's and young people's settings

What you will learn in this unit

- The key areas of health and safety related to work settings.
- Employers' and workers' responsibilities for health and safety.
- Health and safety training required in the work setting.
- Risk assessments in relation to health and safety.
- The importance of protecting the safety and security of all individuals in the work setting.
- Accidents and illness that may take place in work settings and who might deal with them.
- How infection is spread in the workplace.
- Ways to reduce the spread of infection in health, social care and children's and young people's settings.

Important words

Employer – Someone or an organisation that pays workers for their work

Employee – Workers

COSHH – The law linking to the **C**ontrol of **S**ubstances that are **H**azardous to **H**ealth

Procedures – Steps to take when doing a task

First aider – Someone with a first aid qualification

Safe disposal – To throw away safely

Evacuate – Leave a building or area safely

1.1 1.2 1.3 Key areas and responsibilities for health and safety related to the work setting

When working in health, social care and children's and young people's settings, it is very important to work in a way that keeps everyone safe and healthy. Organisations (employers) need to have written procedures which contain rules about how to work safely and these must be checked regularly to make sure that they will support a safe working environment. Organisations must provide equipment and training needed to keep everyone safe.

Workers (employees) must always follow all of the setting procedures so that they work in a way that keeps themselves and others safe. They must always use the protective equipment available in the work setting.

There are seven key areas of health and safety that we need to know about.

Fire safety

All organisations need to have a plan in case of fire. This plan will include how to get out of a building quickly and safely. There has to be a clearly signed exit route out of the building and it is law that these exits are kept clear and the doors can be opened easily in the event of a fire.

It is also part of the law that **firefighting equipment** such as fire extinguishers and fire blankets are kept in good working order. Most settings will have fire alarm systems that must be tested regularly so that in the event of a fire, a loud alarm will warn people to evacuate the building quickly.

Settings will have regular fire evacuation practices so that in the event of a real fire, everyone will know how to get out of the building quickly and safely. All fire evacuations, whether real or just practices, must be recorded.

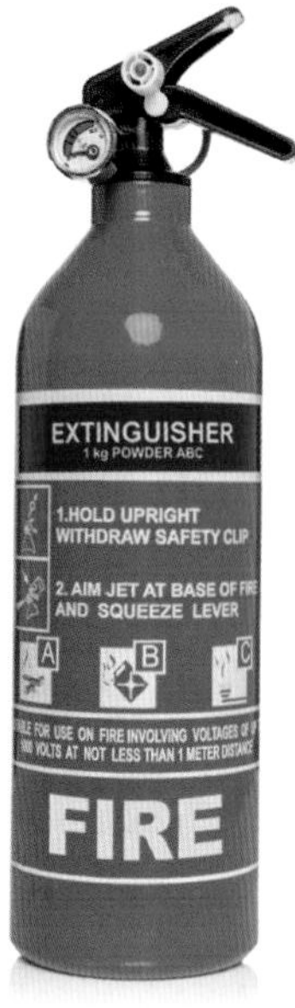

Figure 6.1

Moving and handling

When working with children, people with illness, physical disability or older aged adults, a care worker may need to help them to move around. It is important that this is done in a way that does not cause any injury or pain to the person being moved or to the care worker. Therefore, organisations must make sure that workers know how to move people around safely. **Special equipment** and training on how to use this equipment and how to move people safely must be provided by organisations so that care workers know how to move people around safely.

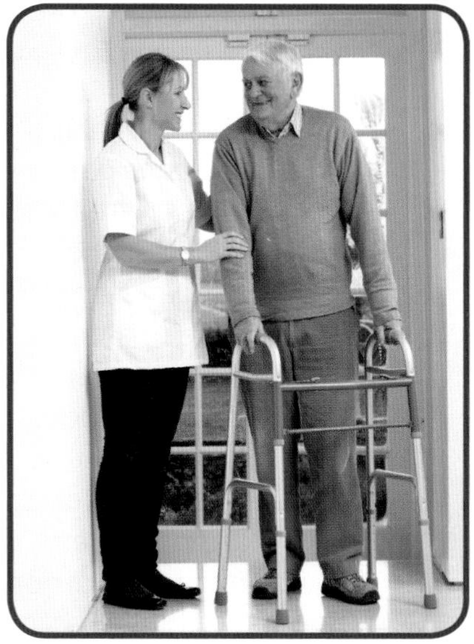

Figure 6.2 A care worker helping an older person

First aid

Accidents do happen, so it is very important that if a child or an adult has an accident, they can be helped quickly and safely. Every organisation must make sure that some or all of the care workers have a first aid qualification so if an accident happens, the person who is hurt can quickly receive the right care and treatment. First aiders must make sure that they work in a way that keeps them and the injured person safe. This means wearing **protective clothing and gloves** if they are dealing with blood.

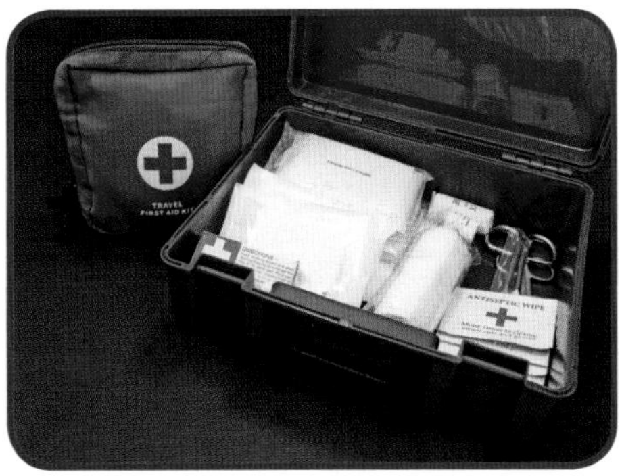

Figure 6.3 A first aid box

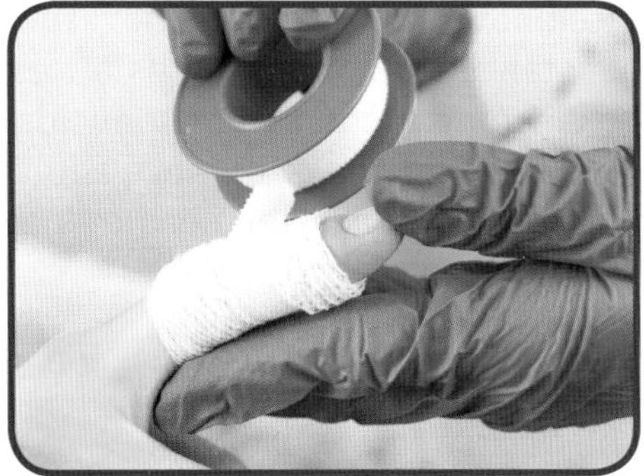

Figure 6.4 Protective gloves

First aiders will know when it is right to treat a person themselves because the injury is not serious, but they will also understand when the injury is serious and it is necessary to get medical help quickly.

The first aider must record all accidents that happen in an accident book and this must be signed by the first aider and the person who is injured. If a child is injured, then the parents must be informed and asked to sign the accident book.

Security

All organisations must know who is in the building at all times; this includes care workers, people using the services and visitors. When they arrive at the work setting, care workers usually have to sign in using a register, code or swipe card. Organisations are required to make sure that everyone is safe, so doors to a setting, such as a care home or nursery, will be locked so that children and vulnerable adults are not able to walk out on their own. It is usual for organisations to have a visitors book that must be signed when someone visits the setting.

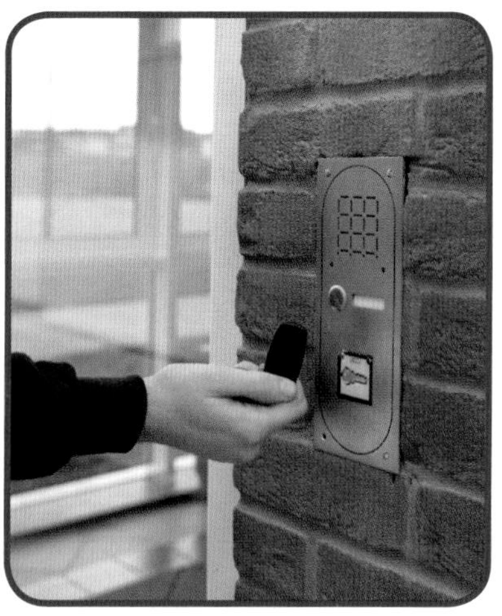

Figure 6.5 Swipe entry system

Storage and disposal of hazardous substances

Care organisations or care workers often have to use or store hazardous substances. Hazardous substances can be cleaning products or chemicals used in the care and treatment of adults and children, such as used needles, nappy waste and blood products.

It is the law (COSHH) that all organisations must store hazardous substances safely, use them in a safe way, and then dispose of them safely. All chemicals must be stored in a locked cupboard that is only opened by people allowed to do so. When chemicals are brought into a setting, there has to be a risk assessment. The assessment will give instructions on how to use the chemicals safely and also give instructions on what to do if the chemicals are spilled or used incorrectly.

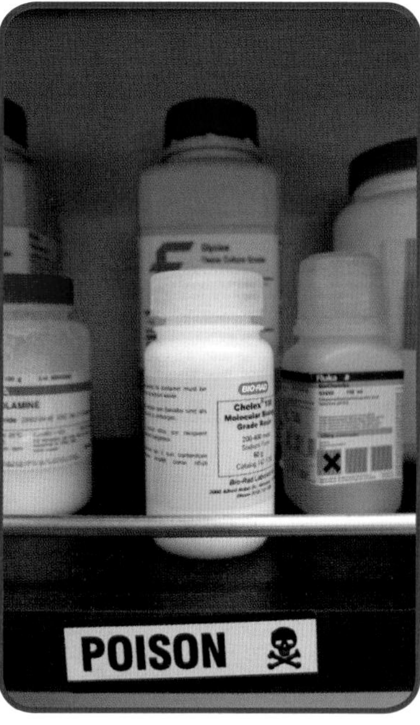

Figure 6.6 Hazardous substances

Records must be kept to show that any hazardous waste has been disposed of safely, for example, by use of a special bin collection service.

Medication storage and administration

When organisations or care workers have to store and give medication to children and adults, there are very strict rules to follow. This is because if medicines are given to the wrong person, or the wrong amount is given to an adult or child, it could cause them serious harm or even death.

Organisations must provide locked storage cupboards and make a record of all medicines that are stored. When medicines are given to adults, this must be done by a qualified person such as a nurse or care worker, and they must record the time and amount given. When giving medicines prescribed by a doctor, nursery workers in a setting must have written permission from the parent or carer before they are able to give the child the medicine. All medicines given to children must also be recorded and the record signed by the nursery nurse and the parent.

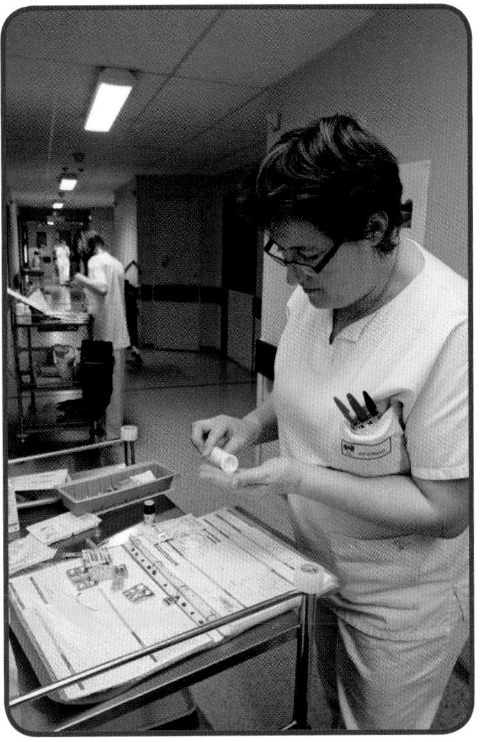

Figure 6.7 Nurse dispensing medicines

Infection prevention and control

All organisations must have policies and procedures which show that the prevention and control of infection has been thought about carefully. Procedures are steps which must be followed by everyone, such as:

- Hand washing procedures – Warm water and soap are always available and hand drying is carried out properly to try and reduce the spread of germs and infection.
- Nappy changing procedures – **Protective aprons and gloves** are used and the area well cleaned after every nappy change to stop the spread of any infection. Nappies and cleaning cloths must be disposed of in a special bin.

- Needle disposal procedures – All used needles must be placed in a special bin where they cannot be removed. When full, the bin is taken away by a registered waste disposal company.
- Body fluids procedures – Vomit, urine, faeces and blood are all body products which can contain germs and infection; therefore, they must be cleaned up and disposed of in a controlled way **using protective clothing**, separate cleaning equipment and special waste bins.

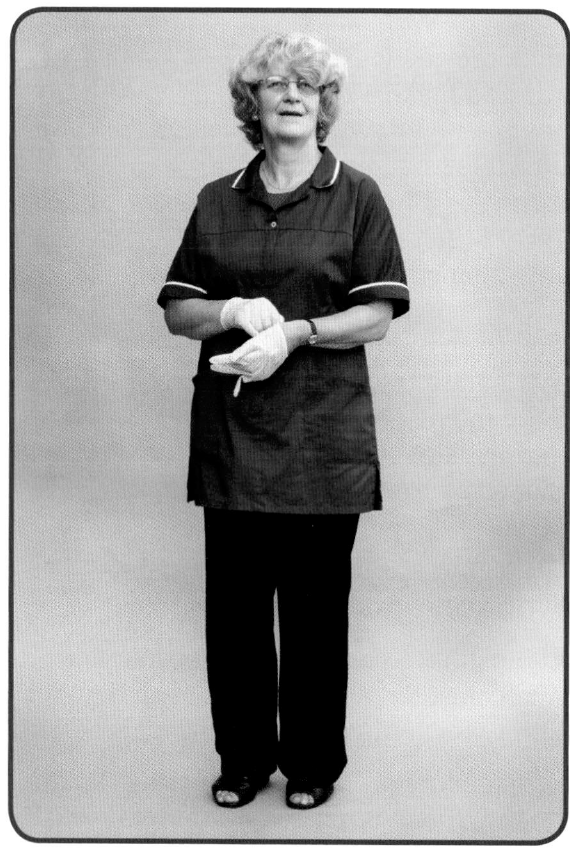

Figure 6.8 A carer wearing protective clothing

1.4 Health and safety training required in the work setting

All workers in health, social care and children's and young people's settings will need to have some health and safety training. This could include:

- training to learn about setting policies and procedures and how to follow them correctly
- first aid training

- safe moving and handling training
- COSSH (hazardous substance) training
- fire evacuation training.

Assessment task 1.1 1.2 1.3 1.4

You have just got a job in a day nursery or care home.

- What key areas of health and safety do you need to know about?
- What are your responsibilities as a worker, for health and safety?
- What are the employer's responsibilities for health and safety?
- What health and safety training will you need?
- When should you use personal protective equipment?

2.1 2.2 Hazards and risks

A hazard is something that can cause injury or harm to a person or group of people. A risk is what can happen as the result of a hazard. For example:

Hazard	Risk
A tray with cups left on the stairs in a care home	People tripping over the tray and falling on the stairs
The soiled nappy bin	If left open, young children might put their hands into the bin and develop an infection
The chemical storage cupboard	
Doors to the setting	If left unlocked, children and vulnerable adults may go out alone
Trailing wires and cables	

Table 6.1 Examples of hazards and risks

Assessment task 2.1 2.2

Write down what is meant by risk.

Complete the table above to show examples of hazards and risks.

2.3 Risk assessments

A risk assessment is completed to show where the dangers are in a work setting (the hazard).

The risk assessment will also show what might happen (the risk) if the hazard is not identified.

The risk assessment should show ways to try and get rid of the hazard, or reduce the risk of injury or harm (the control).

The hazard	The risk	The control
Objects left on the stairs in a care home **Figure 6.9**	People tripping over the objects and falling on the stairs	Make sure items are *never* placed on the stairs
Hot drinks **Figure 6.10**	Burns, scalds to children and adults	• Never carry hot drinks around a work setting • Always place hot drinks on a work surface in the staff area • Hot drinks should be at a safe temperature before being served to others

Table 6.2 Example of a risk assessment

2.4 Know when a risk assessment needs to be carried out

A risk assessment should be carried out and checked regularly to make sure that a work setting is safe for everyone. A risk assessment should also be carried out when:

- A child or adult has different needs (such as a wheelchair user).
- New equipment is brought into the work setting.
- New staff join the setting.
- An accident happens in the work setting.
- It has been six months since the last risk assessment was carried out.

Assessment task 2.3 2.4

Make a health and safety poster which tells new staff about the importance of risk assessments and when a risk assessment should be carried out.

3.1 The importance of protecting your own security and the security of others in the work setting

It is the law that all workers protect themselves and others in the work setting. This can be done by always following work setting procedures. By following procedures, tasks are always carried out in the safest way. Workers who do their job properly, by always following procedures correctly, keep themselves safe and secure. This is because if there is an accident or something goes wrong in the setting, and all procedures have been followed, they will not be to blame. If workers do not follow procedures correctly and something goes wrong, they are breaking the law and may lose their job.

3.2 The importance of safe moving and handling

When working in health, social care and children's and young people's settings, people and equipment must be moved safely, so that no one is injured. Care workers may need to help older aged adults to get out of bed, or help them into the bath, so it is important that they have training to do this safely. Nursery workers will need to safely lift babies and young children in and out of highchairs and cots.

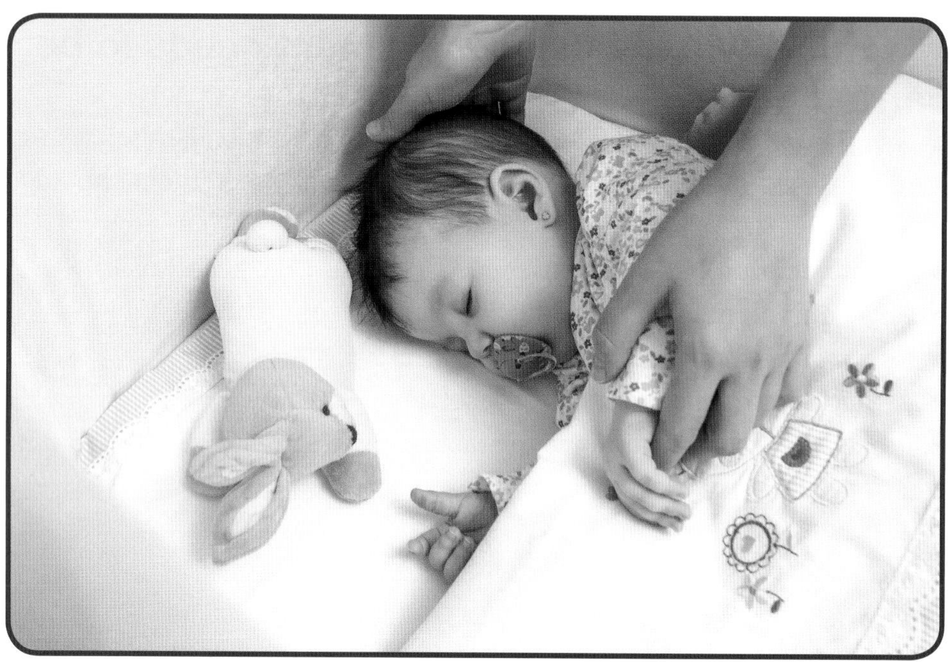

Figure 6.11 Nursery workers need proper training to safely handle children

Work settings will provide the training but it is the responsibility of the care worker to always carry out moving and handling in the correct way. This is important because if they try to save time or do not use equipment properly, they could cause harm or injury to themselves or the people they are caring for.

Assessment task 3.1 3.2

Make a leaflet for nursery workers showing why it is important to protect themselves and others in the work setting by always following procedures.

On the leaflet say why it is important to always follow safe moving and handling procedures.

3.3 3.4 Accidents and illness that may take place in work settings and who might deal with them

When an accident happens in a setting, it must always be reported to the first aider who will deal with the injured child or adult. If everyone in the setting is first aid trained, it will be the first aider who is nearest to the accident who would deal with it.

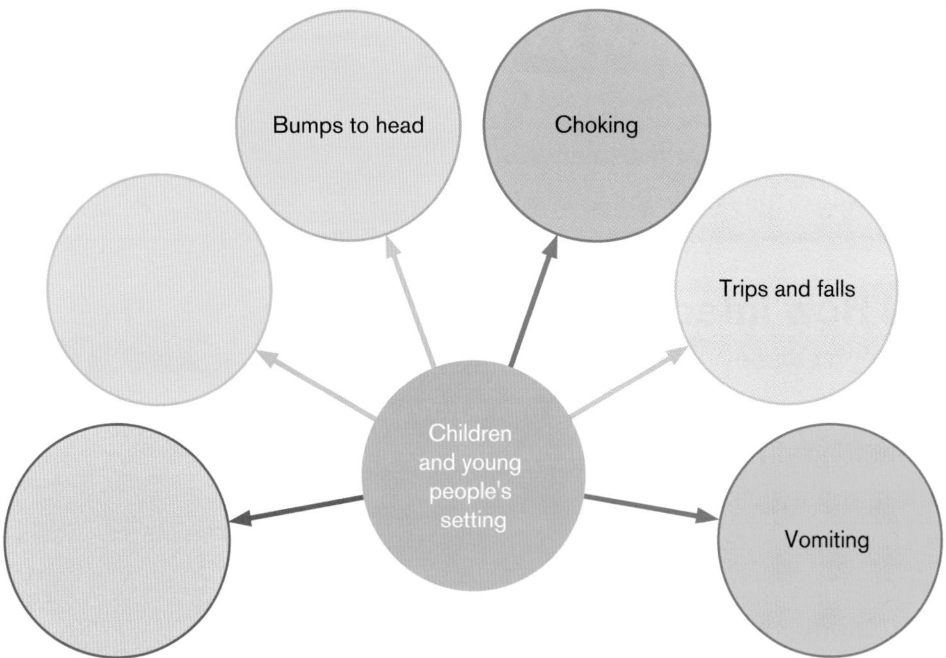

Figure 6.12 Children and young people's setting

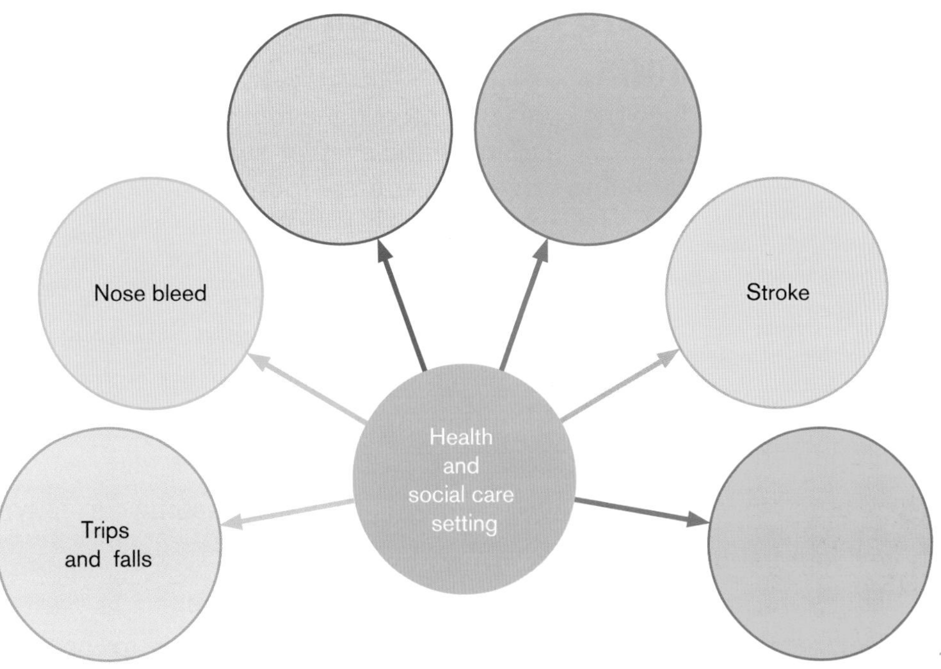

Figure 6.13 Health and social care setting

Assessment task 3.3 3.4

Complete the spider diagrams to show accidents and sudden illness that may occur in both of the settings.

Say who might deal with the accidents and illness.

4.1 How infection is spread in the workplace

Infection can be spread in many ways. A few of these ways include:

- not following hand washing procedures
- not following disposal of body fluid procedures
- sharing towels
- sharing feeding equipment
- not cleaning toys properly
- attending the setting when unwell or with an infection
- unclean surfaces.

4.2 Ways to reduce the spread of infection in health, social care and children's and young people's settings

The best way to reduce the spread of infection is to make sure that there is a high standard of cleanliness and everyone in the setting follows all of the health and safety procedures. Young children and some adults will need to be supported to carry out procedures properly such as hand washing or toileting.

4.3 The standard methods of washing hands

Correct hand washing is the best way to prevent the spread of infection in a setting. So it is very important that everyone washes and dries their hands properly.

There are five steps that need to be followed in hand washing correctly:

1 Wet your hands using clean warm water.
2 Using soap, lather your hands by rubbing them together.
3 Clean between the fingers and under your nails, scrubbing to the count of ten.
4 Rinse hands well in clean, running water.
5 Dry hands well using an air dryer or separate hand towel.

Source: **www.uhb.nhs.uk/Downloads/pdf/HandHygienePoster.pdf**

Assessment task 4.1 4.2 4.3

Make an information poster to put up in a care home, showing:

- how infection can be spread
- ways to reduce the spread of infection
- the best way to hand wash properly.

Summary

In this unit you have learned that:

- There are key areas of health and safety related to work settings.
- Employers and workers have responsibilities for health and safety.
- Health and safety training is required in the work setting.
- Risk assessments are used in relation to health and safety.
- It is important to protect the safety and security of all individuals in the work setting.
- Accidents and illness may take place in work settings and there are people who are trained to deal with them.
- Infection can spread in the workplace if procedures are not followed correctly.
- There are ways to reduce the spread of infection in health, social care and children's and young people's settings.

Chapter 7

PWCS 05 Introductory awareness of person-centred support in health, social care and children's and young people's settings

What you will learn in this unit

- What is meant by person-centred support.
- The benefits of person-centred support.
- How to provide person-centred support.
- How individuals can be in control of their care needs.
- How risk assessments can assist person-centred support.

Important words

Life event – Something that has happened to a person that has affected their life, such as serious illness or loss of a family member

Assessing risk – Seeing things that might be a danger to someone

Assist – Help

Safety control – Things that can be done to reduce the risk of injury

1.1 What is person-centred support?

Person-centred support is about putting the needs and wishes of a person first. This is done by listening to a person and understanding the importance of meeting their individual needs, in a way that is right for them.

This is very different to not giving person-centred support, where a service may be offered, even if it does not meet all of the person's needs.

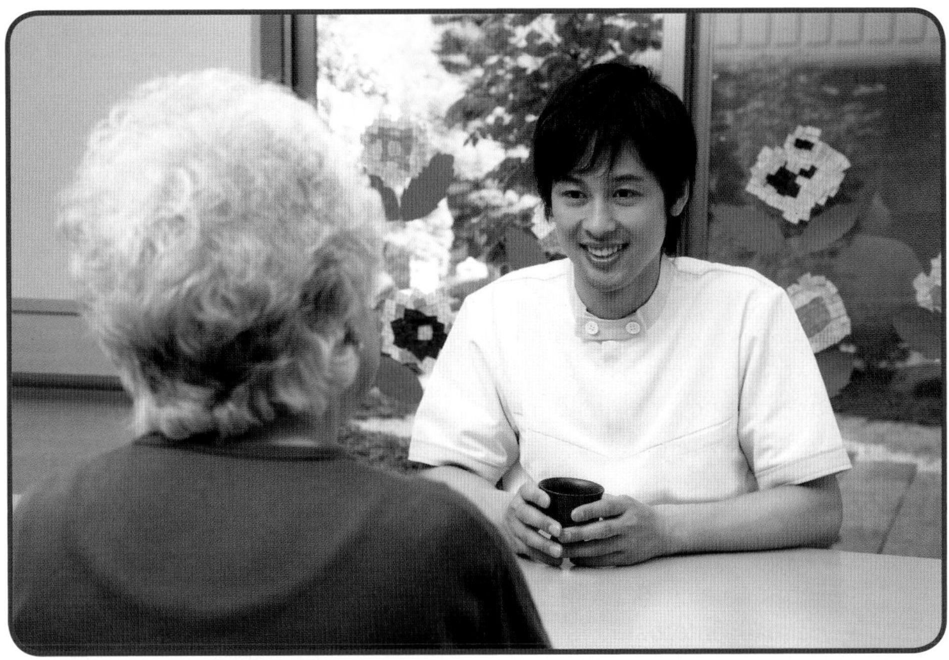

Figure 7.1 Care worker talking to an adult

1.2 Outline the importance of finding out an individual's history, needs, wishes, likes and dislikes

It is very important to ask children and adults about their wishes, likes and dislikes so that you understand what care and support would be best for them. It is also very important to find out about a person's history (this could be their medical history or a life event) so that the person can be supported in a sensitive and effective way.

Sometimes people are not able to tell you what they want or need, so you will need to communicate with others who may have this information, such as family members, parents, nursery or care workers.

If time is not taken to get this important information about a person's history, needs, wishes, likes and dislikes, the wrong help might be offered or the person may not feel their needs are being met. This could make them feel unhappy, lonely, worried or even unwell.

Assessment task 1.1 1.2

Define person-centred support

Using the scenario below, outline the importance of finding out about Ben's history, needs, wishes, likes and dislikes.

Scenario

Ben is two years old and will be starting nursery soon. Ben's mum is a little worried about him starting nursery as up to now he has only been cared for by family members. She wants Ben to be happy and stay healthy when he is at nursery. Ben has had a few health problems and is allergic to all milk products. Ben is not really interested in listening to stories or playing with jigsaws, but loves to be outdoors climbing and riding on sit-on toys. Ben's mum has started potty training Ben, but he still has a few accidents during the day.

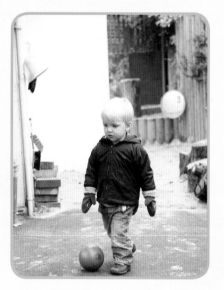

Figure 7.2

1.3 How to provide person-centred support when supporting individuals in day-to-day activities

By using **person-centred practice**, the needs and choices of an individual person are seen as very important. A care worker providing care for an older aged adult in the home should take the time to find out about their needs and wishes. This means that they can support the individual in their care routine in a way that best suits them. For example, helping the individual to shower in the morning rather than the evening as that is what they would prefer.

Child-centred practice is the same as person-centred practice. This is when the individual care and learning needs of a child are met in a way that is best for them. It is good practice to ask a child about their interests, likes and dislikes when planning activities so that their ideas can be included. For example, if a child is interested in dinosaurs, an activity could be planned to include dinosaurs.

Assessment task 1.3

Discuss person-centred practice in groups and write down more examples of how to provide person-centred support when supporting individuals in day-to-day activities.

2.1 The benefits of person-centred support

When person-centred support is given, the individual will feel valued and respected because they will know that their opinions and wishes are being listened to. This will help them to feel in control of what is happening in their lives. They may feel more confident about making choices and may feel more able to do things for themselves.

Example!

An example of person-centred support

Derek, aged 72, has had a mild stroke and needs some help to get dressed. Norma, his carer, knows that if she gives Derek a little more time to get dressed, he can do most of it on his own. It would be quicker for Norma to dress Derek herself, but she understands that Derek wants to be as independent as possible and do things for himself if he can. By giving Derek this person-centred support, he is able to complete tasks for himself so feels valued and confident.

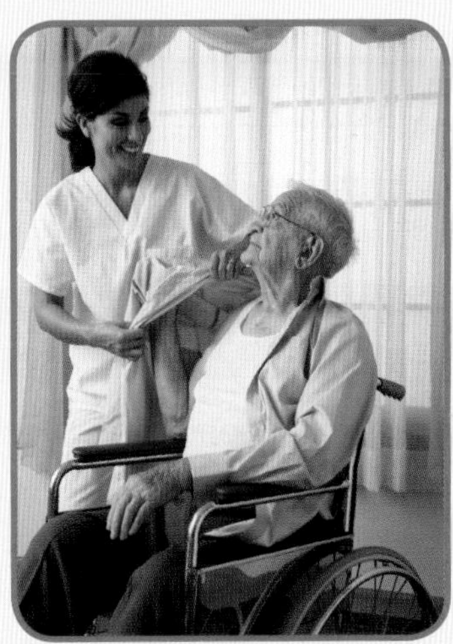

Figure 7.3

2.2 How individuals can be in control of their own care needs

It is important that individuals are supported to be in control of their own care needs. This is mostly done through individuals making their own decisions or being given suitable choices.

Look at the table below and decide how individuals can be supported to take control of their care needs.

Care need	Ways to support children and adults to be in control of their care needs
Maintain body temperature	Choice of wearing more clothing to keep warm or, where possible, turning up the heating Choice of removing a jumper or opening a window if they feel too warm
Sleep and rest	
Suitable clothes – dress and undress	
Personal hygiene	
Food and drink	
Fresh air and exercise	Children should be supervised so that they can choose to play indoors or outdoors Older aged adults can be given a choice of activities such as swimming or walking in the garden

Table 7.1 Ways to support children and adults to be in control of their care needs

Assessment task 2.1 2.2

Discuss other benefits for Derek of being given person-centred support.

Fill in the gaps in the table above to show other ways to allow individuals to be control of their care needs.

2.3 How assessing risk can assist person-centred support

If there are many risks in the environment, it is more likely that a person will come to harm. It is important to look at the environment and where possible, reduce the chance of a child or adult being injured or harmed. This is done through assessing the risks and putting safety controls in place to try to remove as many risks as possible.

For example, if the water temperature in a care home is controlled so that tap water is never too hot, then residents can take a bath when they want to, without needing to have a carer to check that the water is at the right temperature. This will give the resident more independence in their care routines and allows them to have some control to make choices.

By having low sinks and toilets in a day nursery, children who want to use the bathroom independently can do so safely, without having to be taken by a childcare worker. This allows the child to be in control of their own care needs and supports their growing independence. This is an example of child-centred support.

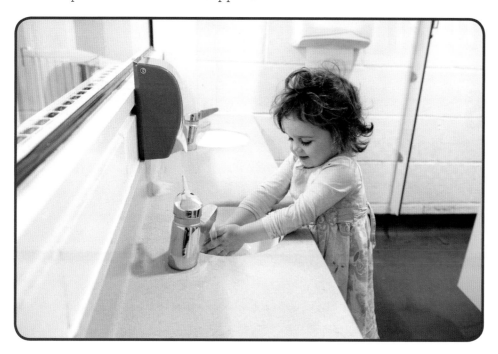

Figure 7.4 Low sinks and toilets support a child's growing independence

Assessment task 2.3

Discuss another way that assessing risk might assist person-centred support.

Summary

In this unit you have learned that:

- There are many benefits of person-centred support.
- There are many ways to give person-centred support.
- Person-centred support helps individuals to be in control of their care needs.
- Risk assessments can assist person-centred support.

Part 2 Optional units

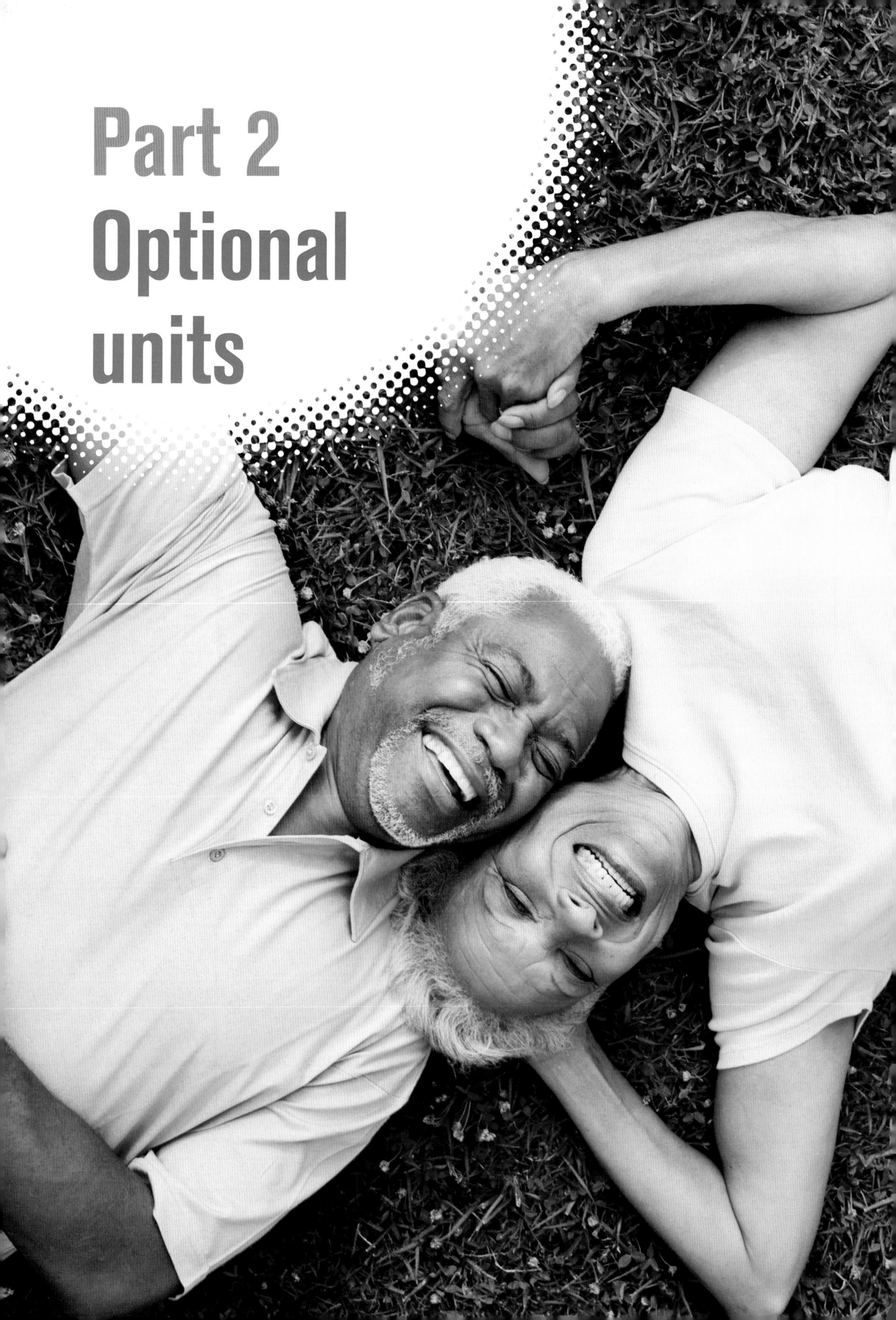

Chapter 8

PWCS 06 Introductory awareness of working with others in health, social care and children's and young people's settings

What you will learn in this unit

- The importance of working with others in health, social care and children's and young people's settings.
- Ways of working with others.
- Ways of working with others that work well.
- Ways of working with others that do not work well.
- The meaning and benefits of partnership working.

Important words

Team work – This is when people work well together

1.1 The importance of working with others

In health, social care and children's and young people's settings, there are many different services offered, such as health care, childcare or homecare services. There are a wide range of people and professionals, with different skills, who work hard to provide these services. Each one of these people has an important job to do, but they could not do their job well without working with other people.

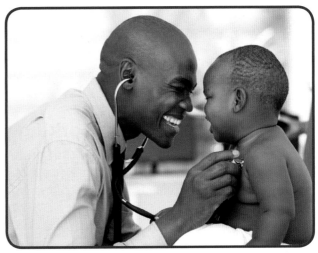

Figure 8.1

There are many services offered in a health centre, for example. Doctors, health visitors, nurses, care workers and dieticians all work together to keep everyone in the community as healthy as possible.

As well as health care professionals, there are other workers, such as cooks, cleaners and office staff who have different jobs.

Example!

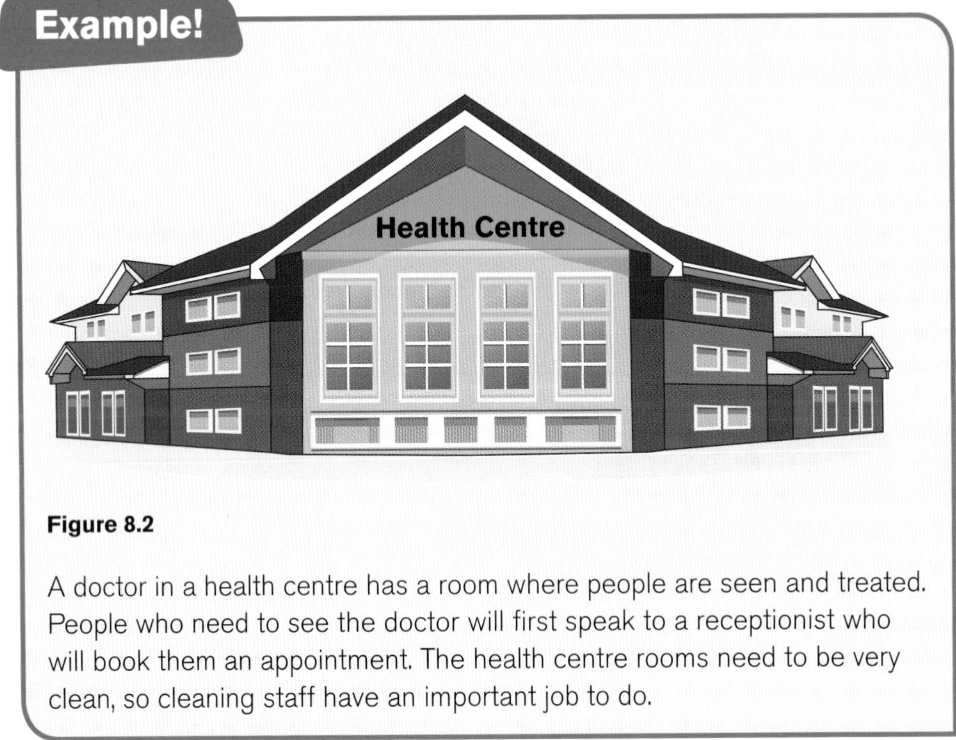

Figure 8.2

A doctor in a health centre has a room where people are seen and treated. People who need to see the doctor will first speak to a receptionist who will book them an appointment. The health centre rooms need to be very clean, so cleaning staff have an important job to do.

It is important that all professionals and others with different jobs to do work together, so that they can provide the very best service.

1.2 Ways of working with others

There are many ways that professionals and others can work together to make sure that the people using the service are well cared for and the service is the best that it can be.

Sharing ideas
Knowing what skills others in the team have
Listening to each other
Using good communication
Sharing information
Offering support and advice
Having meetings
Understanding the importance of teamwork
Ways that professionals and others can work together

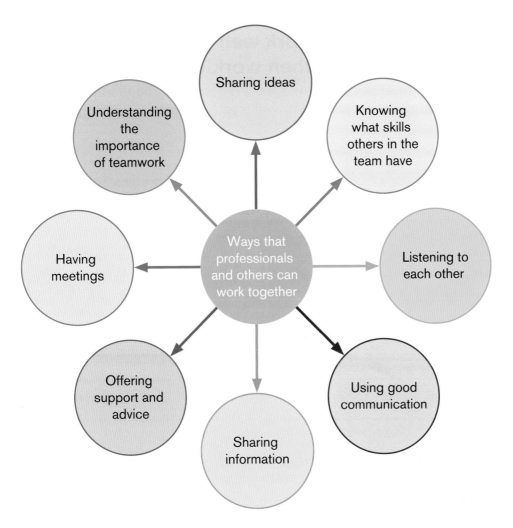

Figure 8.3 Ways of working together

Assessment task 1.1 1.2

Make a noticeboard about working with others:

- say why it is important to work with others
- write down some ways to work with others.

1.3 1.4 Ways that work well and ways that do not work well when working with others

Some things that people do, and the ways that they do them, can mean the difference between working well together and not working well together.

In the table below are examples of this.

Ways that work well when working with others	Ways that do not work well when working with others
Listening to what people say and trying to see their point of view	Listening to others' ideas but not taking any notice of their point of view
Going to meetings and sharing ideas	Going to meetings and not sharing your ideas
Getting to work on time and being reliable	Being late and not letting others know where you are
Speaking clearly and using appropriate language	Not speaking clearly and using slang
Offering support and help	Not helping when someone is struggling
Asking for advice when you need it	Doing everything your own way even if you could work better with help from others

Table 8.1

Assessment task 1.3 1.4

Add information to your noticeboard about:

- ways that work well when working with others
- ways that do not work well when working with others.

2.1 2.2 The meaning of partnership working and examples of who partners may be

Partnership working is when people from different settings or with different skills come together to support individuals or share ideas to solve problems.

Partnership working can take place between workers in a setting or with other professionals who work outside of the setting. Sometimes different settings may work together in partnership to share equipment, staff and ideas.

Example!

A young child in a nursery with a speech and language difficulty may have the support of a speech therapist who comes into the nursery to support the child. The speech therapist will also share ideas with the nursery staff so they understand how best to support the child. The speech therapist and the nursery staff will meet regularly with the child's parents or carers to share information about the child's progress.

Partners in health, social care and children's and young people's settings could include:

- nursery workers
- care workers
- doctors
- health visitors
- speech therapists
- occupational therapists
- receptionists
- cleaning staff
- school nurses
- teachers
- special educational needs co-ordinators.

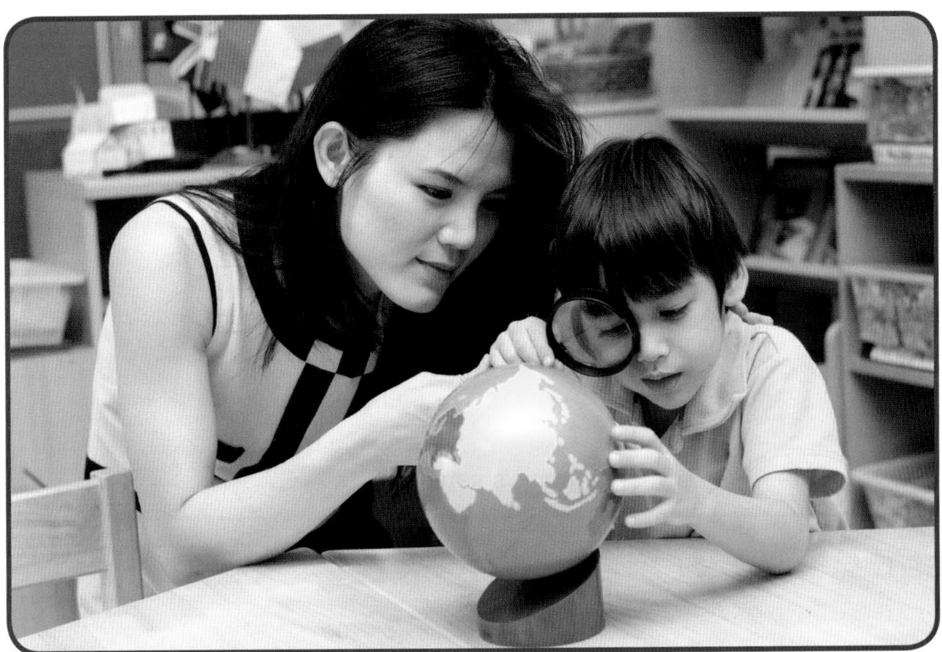

Figure 8.4

2.3 The benefits of partnership working

As mentioned earlier in this chapter, there are many benefits of partnership working in health, social care and children's and young people's settings and these include:

- the correct support being available
- people being seen and treated sooner
- skills being shared
- information being shared appropriately
- equipment being shared
- staff sharing ideas
- professionals learning new skills from each other
- watching the way others work and learning from this.

Assessment task 2.1 2.2 2.3

Add information to your noticeboard about:

- what partnership working means
- who partners might be
- the benefits of partnership working.

Summary

In this unit you have learned that:

- It is important to work with others in health, social care and children's and young people's settings.
- There are many ways of working with others.
- There are some ways of working with others that work well.
- There are some ways of working with others that do not work well.
- There are many benefits of partnership working in health, social care and children's and young people's settings.

Chapter 9

PWCS 07 **Introductory awareness of the importance of healthy eating and drinking for adults**

What you will learn in this unit

- The importance of healthy eating.
- What is meant by a balanced diet.
- Ways to inform people about the importance of a balanced diet.
- The importance of drinking enough fluids to stay healthy.
- Signs that a person is not drinking enough fluids.
- Ways to encourage individuals to drink enough to stay healthy.

Important words

Balanced diet – Daily food that has the right amount of nutrients for health and growth

Contribute to helping an individual stay healthy – Help a person to stay healthy

Inform individuals – Let people know

Recommended daily fluid intake – The amount of water that experts say we should drink everyday

Nutrients – Are found in food and do an important job to keep the body healthy

Antioxidants – Antioxidants work to reverse the damage that pollution has on the body

Dehydrated – Dried out and thirsty

1.1 1.3 Balanced diets and the ways food can help people stay healthy

The main food groups

For children and young people to grow properly and be healthy, they need to eat a range of healthy foods that contain important nutrients.

This is called a **balanced diet**. Adults should also eat a balanced diet to help them to stay fit and healthy.

To have a balanced diet, everybody should make sure that they eat foods from the five main food groups every day.

The five main food groups are:

- carbohydrates – bread, cereals and potatoes
- proteins – fish, meat and meat alternatives
- vitamins and minerals – fruit and vegetables
- calcium – milk, yoghurt and other dairy products
- a small amount of foods containing fats and sugar.

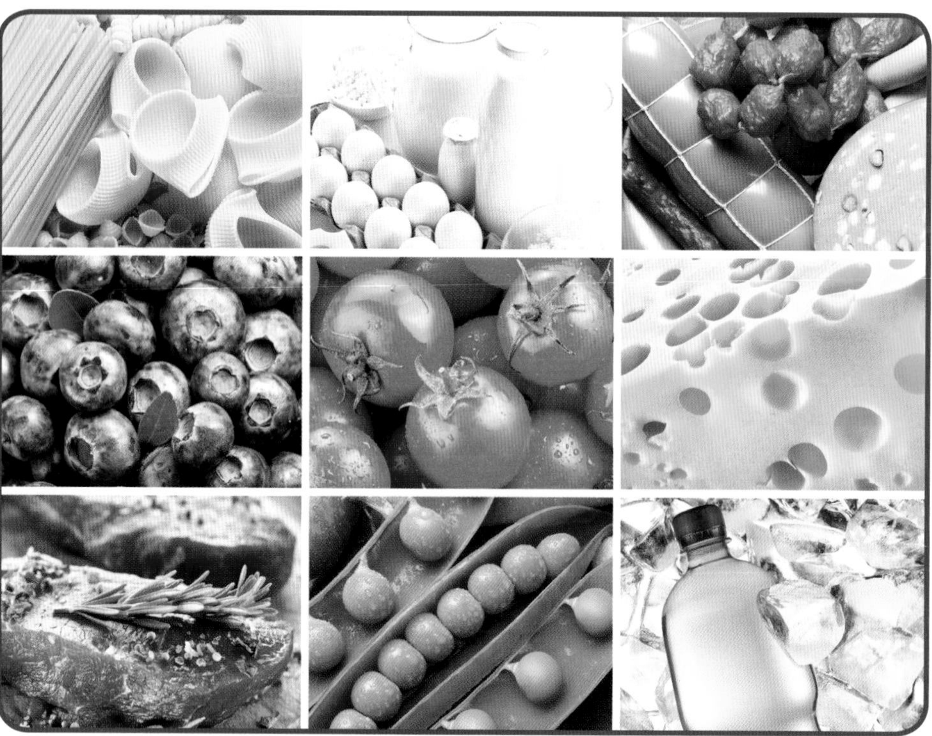

Figure 9.1 Examples of healthy foods

All of the foods from the food groups have benefits for the body and help people to stay fit and healthy.

- **Carbohydrates** give us energy.
- **Proteins** help the body to grow and repair.
- **Vitamins and minerals** help every part of the body to grow and develop so that people have strong bones, healthy teeth, clear skin, healthy heart, etc.
- **Fats** help the body to use all of the fats and minerals where they are needed in the body.

The table below shows all of the main nutrients that make up a balanced diet, the food that these nutrients can be found in and the benefits for the body.

Nutrient	Food the nutrient is found in	Benefits for the body
Protein	Meat, eggs, fish, milk and other dairy products For vegetarians – wheat, oats, pulses, lentils and soya products, such as Quorn burgers	Helps the body to repair cells Helps the body to grow and develop well
Carbohydrates	Bread, pasta, flour, potatoes, couscous and bananas	Gives the body energy Can help to cut the risk of diseases like diabetes and heart disease
Fats	Butter, margarine, vegetable oil, other dairy products and fish	Gives the body energy Helps to build healthy cells Helps to keep our brain healthy
Iron	Red meat, broccoli, spinach, egg yolk, plain chocolate and dried fruits	Helps the blood to carry oxygen through the body During pregnancy the mother's iron helps the baby's brain to develop
Calcium	Milk, cheese, butter, yoghurt, other dairy products, cereals and grains	Good for healthy bones and teeth Helps to keep our hearts healthy
Vitamin A	Carrots, milk, apricots, oily fish and margarine	Good for healthy eyes and clear eyesight
Vitamin B	Bread, meat, pasta, flour, rice, noodles and yeast	Good for a healthy nervous system Helps the body to release energy from other food
Vitamin C	Oranges, lemons, grapefruits, blackcurrants, kiwis, potatoes and sweet potatoes	Good for healthy gums and skin Helps to heal cuts Can help treat the common cold
Vitamin E	Vegetable oil, spinach, nuts and wheat germ	Works as an antioxidant, protecting the eyes, liver and skin from environmental pollution

Table 9.1 The main nutrients in a balanced diet, the food groups these nutrients are found in and the benefits for the body

1.2 The effects on health if a diet is not balanced

If individuals do not eat a balanced diet and do not eat enough of the healthy, nutritious food shown in the table above, their bodies may not develop properly or they may have health problems. If individuals eat too much unhealthy food, like fast or junk food, they may feel a lack of energy, become obese or develop illness and disease.

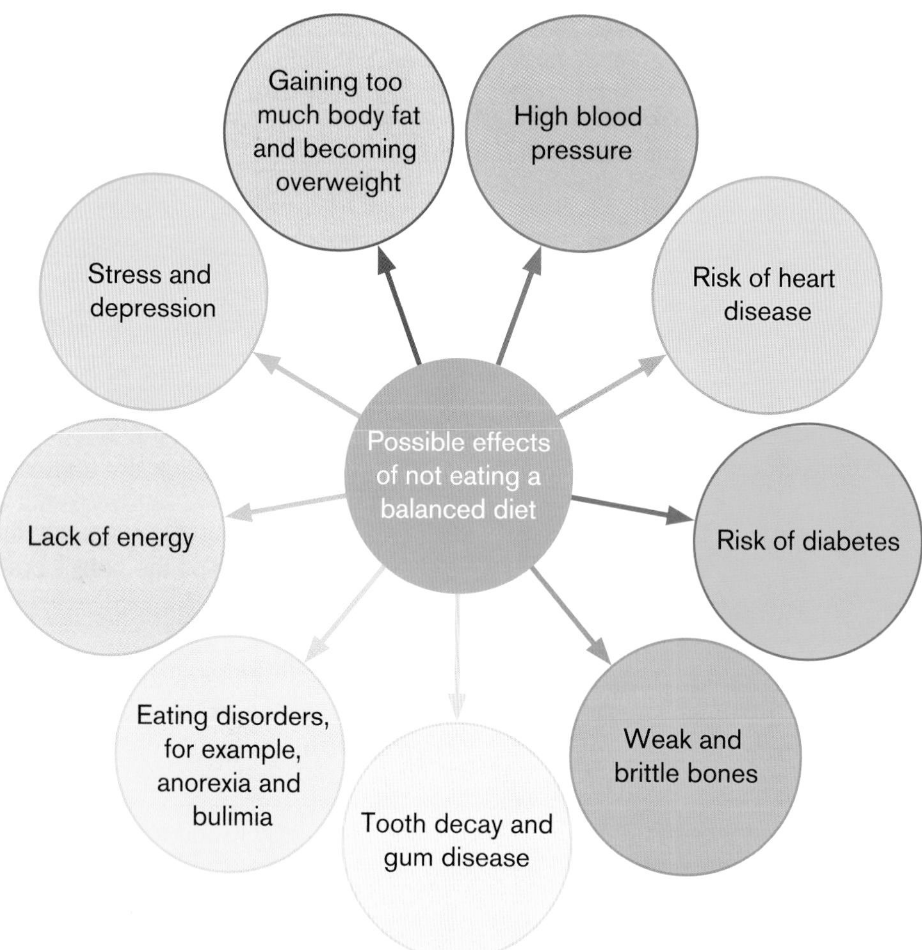

Figure 9.2 Possible effects of not eating a balanced diet

Assessment task 1.1 1.2 1.3

Design a leaflet that can be given out at the local doctor's surgery that shows:

- what is meant by a balanced diet
- the effects on health if a diet is not balanced
- ways that food can contribute to helping an individual to stay healthy.

1.4 Ways to inform people to eat a balanced diet

Some people do not understand the importance of eating a balanced diet, perhaps because they have never learned about healthy eating or because they do not understand the dangers of eating a poor diet. This means that informing people about the benefits of eating a healthy diet is very important, so they are healthy and happy.

Ways that people can be informed about healthy diets are:

- researching on the internet
- reading books, magazines and leaflets
- getting advice from health care workers or nutritionists
- joining a club or group interested in healthy weight
- being aware of nutrition tables on food packages.

Assessment task 1.4

Make a poster to outline the ways that individuals can get information about eating a balanced diet.

2.1 2.2 The recommended daily fluid intake and how drinking enough can help you to stay healthy

The human body needs enough water and other fluids to stay healthy, work properly and not become dehydrated. Water is not just important for stopping us feeling thirsty; we also need water to make our cells work properly. Water also has the job of carrying the important nutrients around the body in the blood and taking away the waste products from our body. It is important for people to drink water and other healthy drinks all through the day to put the fluid back that is lost through sweating, passing urine and even breathing. Sugary, fizzy drinks and alcohol are not healthy fluids and these types of drinks will make the body lose water and become dehydrated.

Health professionals suggest that:

- Women should drink around 1.5 litres of fluid every day (8 glasses).
- Men should drink around 2 litres of fluid every day (10 glasses).

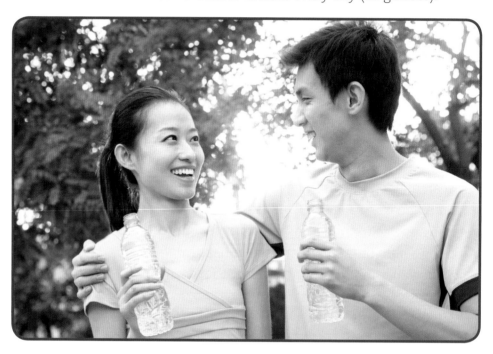

Figure 9.3 It is important for people to drink water throughout the day

2.3 2.4 The signs of not drinking enough and how this can affect health

There are signs that people can feel and see when they are not drinking enough healthy fluids and have become dehydrated.

Not needing to go to the toilet very often and passing dark coloured urine when they go
Getting headaches
Feeling dizzy or lightheaded
Not having very much energy
Dry mouth and lips
Sunken eyes
Fast heartbeat
Feeling short-tempered
Cold hands and feet

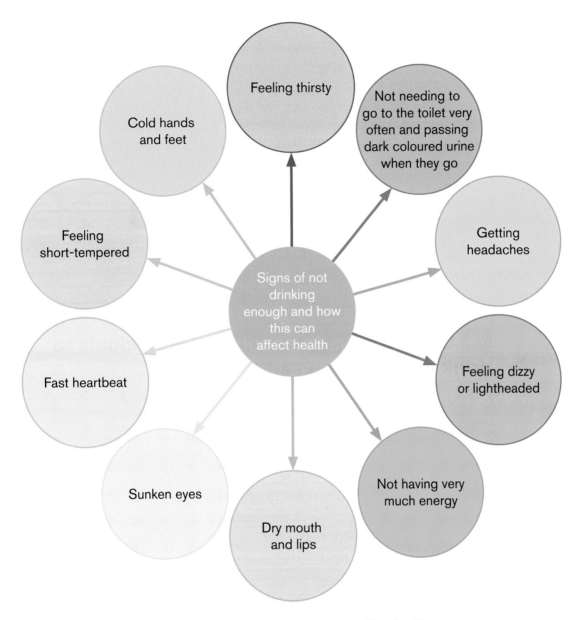

Figure 9.4 Signs of not drinking enough and how this can affect health

If dehydration is not treated properly and the lost fluids are not replaced, people can become unwell and if they continue to not drink enough, they may develop long-term illness:

Short- and long-term effects to health of not drinking enough:

- Heat exhaustion – this can be caused by losing water through sweating and not drinking enough to replace the lost fluids
- Liver damage – is caused through not drinking enough fluids
- Kidney problems – kidney stones can grow if a person does not drink enough fluids every day

- Muscle and joint damage – the right levels of fluids in the body are needed to keep muscles and joints working correctly
- Constipation – not being able to empty the bowels of the body's waste due to lack of fluids
- The pulse becomes weak and low blood pressure can also be a problem when a person does have enough fluids in the body
- A person can become unconsciousness and vital organs can begin to shut down when the body is lacking in fluids

Assessment task 2.1 2.2 2.3 2.4

Make a poster to help people to understand the importance of drinking enough to stay healthy. Do some research using books and the internet and include what you have learned in 2.1–2.4 in this unit.

2.5 Outline ways to encourage individuals to drink enough to stay healthy

It is important that everyone drinks enough fluids to stay hydrated and healthy. Some of the ways to encourage children and adults to drink fluids include:

- having easy access to water from taps or water coolers.
- carrying a small bottle of water.
- putting water into child-friendly containers (such as cups with pictures of their favourite characters).
- taking a drink of water to the bedroom to drink during the night.
- offering more drinks during hot weather.
- offering ice lollies to keep cool and hydrated in the summer.
- offer older aged adults regular drinks.
- regularly offer babies cool, boiled water.
- offer a drink with snacks and at meal times.

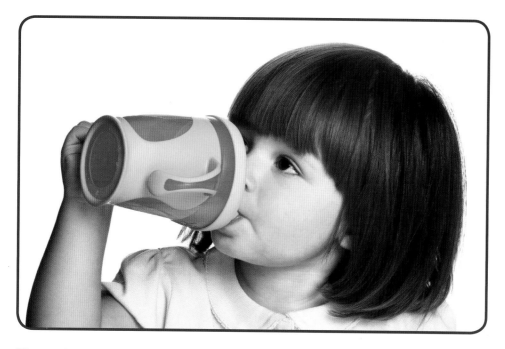

Figure 9.5 Child-friendly water container

Assessment task 2.5

Julie is seven years old and has recently suffered with very dry lips and mouth. The health visitor has suggested that Julie might not be drinking enough fluids. How can Julie's mum encourage her to drink enough fluids to stay healthy?

Summary

In this unit you have learned that:

- Healthy eating is very important to support growth and development.
- A balanced diet is needed to stay healthy.
- All people should understand the importance of a balanced diet.
- People must drink enough fluids to stay healthy.
- There are many signs and symptoms when a person is not drinking enough fluids.
- It is important to encourage individuals to drink enough to stay healthy.

Chapter 10

CFC 15 Human growth and development

What you will learn in this unit

- The stages of growth and development that people go through.
- The factors that may affect physical growth and development.
- The effects of ageing later on in life.

Important words

Well-being – Health

Emotional and social well-being – Happiness in yourself and as part of a group (society)

Pathway – A timeline

Factors – Negative or positive things that may have happened

Circumstances or life events – Situations or experiences in a person's life

Case study

Grace is 82 years old. She lives alone because her husband died two years ago. Grace has lived an active life but has recently suffered a stroke. She has made some good progress and, as she is getting better, she is hoping to leave the hospital soon to go home.

Grace's daughter lives nearby so she will help Grace by making her dinner and doing jobs around the house.

Before Grace is allowed to leave the hospital, a specialist nurse must assess how well Grace will be able to manage at home. She needs to find out about Grace's physical, intellectual, emotional and social well-being.

Grace enjoyed swimming for most of her life, and swam twice a week in the local pool as a child and throughout her life until she reached the age of 74. Grace always made sure that she ate a good balanced diet, but during her teenage years she did admit to smoking for a couple of years. However, she realised it was unhealthy and soon stopped.

She caught measles when she was seven years old which made her very ill. Grace has slight hearing loss in one ear because of this illness.

The happiest times in Grace's life were when she married Bob, her husband, and when her children were born. The time when Grace was most sad was when her husband died; she then had to live alone. Another difficult time for Grace was when she suffered the stroke. This made her very frightened and worried about how she would look after herself in the future.

1.1 Human growth and development

People move through different stages of growth and development during their lives. When we are talking about a person's lifetime, we can look at five important 'life stages', which are shown in Figure 10.1.

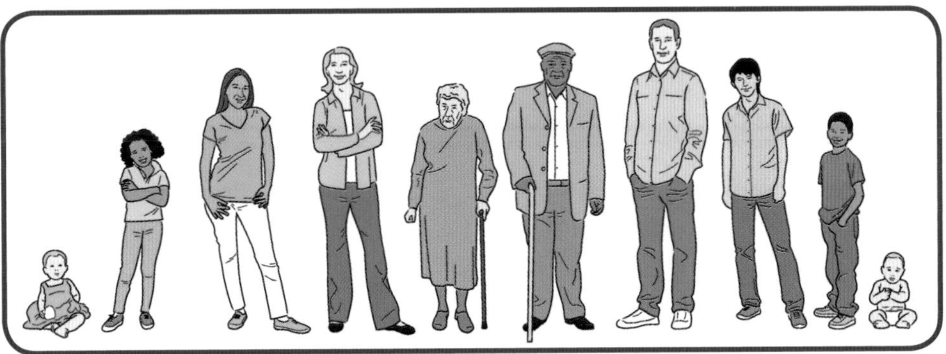

Figure 10.1 Five important life stages

Infancy

This is the time between birth and five years. It is a time when young children need their families to provide everything they need, as they are not able to care for themselves yet. Although most children at this age will not be at school, they are learning at a very fast rate. During this time children change from being a tiny baby to a school-aged child who can walk, talk and begin to care for themselves.

Childhood

This is the time in a child's life when they start full-time school and begin to have their own friends. The stage of childhood begins at the age of five and continues until a child is about 12 years old. Again, growth and development are happening quickly and a child changes a great deal during this stage.

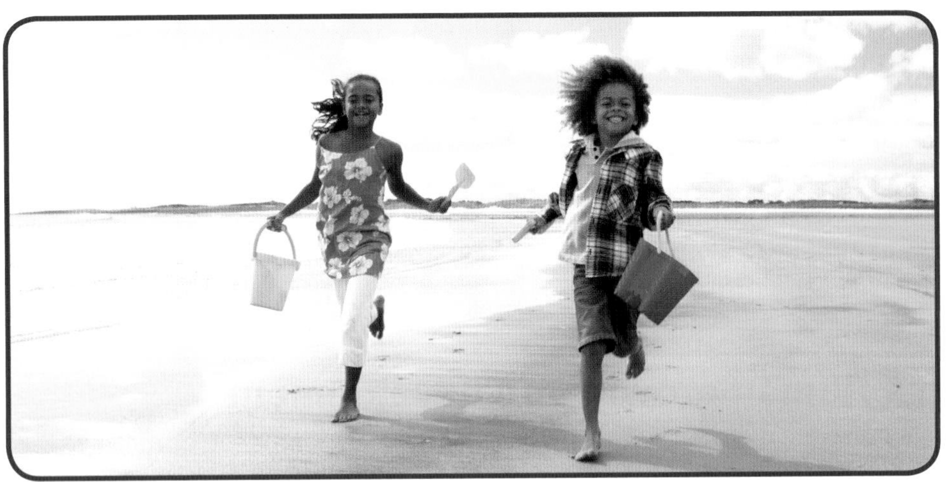

Figure 10.2 Childhood

Adolescence

This stage in a person's life begins at around 12 or 13 years of age, as they become a teenager. During this teenage stage, the body goes through many physical changes which are linked to reproduction (having babies). Hormone changes inside the body can affect growth, mood and appearance. Some teenagers find this stage of their life quite difficult, but most of their teenage worries will have disappeared as they reach adulthood.

Adulthood

When people move into adulthood, they probably have a job, a partner and perhaps even a family of their own to care for. Physical growth and development have stopped, and later in adulthood the body begins to show signs of ageing; for example, a person may not be able to run so fast or climb so many stairs. However, social and emotional changes are still happening at this time and the brain is still working very well.

Older adulthood

During this life stage, people are more likely to become ill or physically less able. This is because a person's body is beginning to wear out, particularly if they did not take care of their bodies when they were teenagers and adults. If we smoke or drink too much alcohol, it could damage our bodies.

During this life stage, skin begins to lose elasticity so will become lined; hair will lose its colour so become grey. Muscles weaken, so walking may become slower and tasks such as taking tight lids off jars may be difficult.

Some older people might have sight or hearing loss. Many older people live alone due to the death of a partner, so may become lonely. Getting out and meeting friends can become more difficult if people are worried about going out alone or when it is dark.

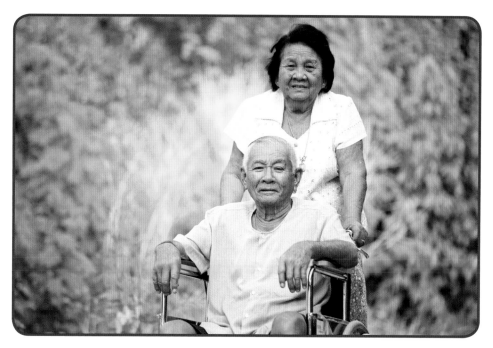

Figure 10.3 Older adulthood brings many challenges

Task!

In small groups, think about an older person that you know (it could be a neighbour or grandparent). Discuss the effects that ageing has had on these people.

Assessment task 1.1 1.2 2.1

Make a poster showing:

- A pathway of Grace's life. Remember to include all five stages: use pictures from magazines or draw what a person at each stage will look like.
- A brief description of the effects of ageing that Grace may have experienced during older adulthood.
- What is meant by physical, intellectual, emotional and social development. Use the information below to help you.

1.2 What is physical, intellectual, emotional and social development?

Physical development

This means the way in which bodies grow and how people develop physical skills. As we move into older adulthood, physical skills or activities may become more difficult. A baby learns to walk, a child learns how to run and jump, a teenager might run quickly and jump over objects, an adult might run even faster; however, as people become much older this might become more difficult. As they age, some older adults may need a stick to support them when walking.

Intellectual development

This is the way in which our brain develops and works. As we go through the different life stages, our brain takes in more information that we can understand and use. However, as we move through older adulthood, the brain may start to slow down and we may become forgetful or confused.

Emotional development

This is the development of lots of emotions, from sad to happy, and excited to angry. During each stage, people have different emotions to deal with; for example, a teenager may worry about exams or friendships, whereas an adult may worry about household bills or the family.

Social development

This is about understanding the needs of others as well as your own, within social relationships. It is about understanding how to behave in different places. For example, children need to understand how to behave towards teachers and their friends in school, and teenagers have different social experiences in college. Older adults might lose partners or friends, and need to find new ways to socialise.

2.1 Factors affecting growth and development

As a person goes through the life stages from birth to older adulthood, there are many factors which may affect physical growth, such as exercise, diet, lifestyle or illness.

Life events which can affect emotional and social well-being

There are also certain times in a person's life that can affect their emotional and social well-being. Good experiences that make an adult feel happy may include a birth in the family, getting married, getting a good job or moving to a nice house. There could also be times in an adult's life when they feel sad or very worried, such as losing a home or a job, a family splitting up or the death of a close family member.

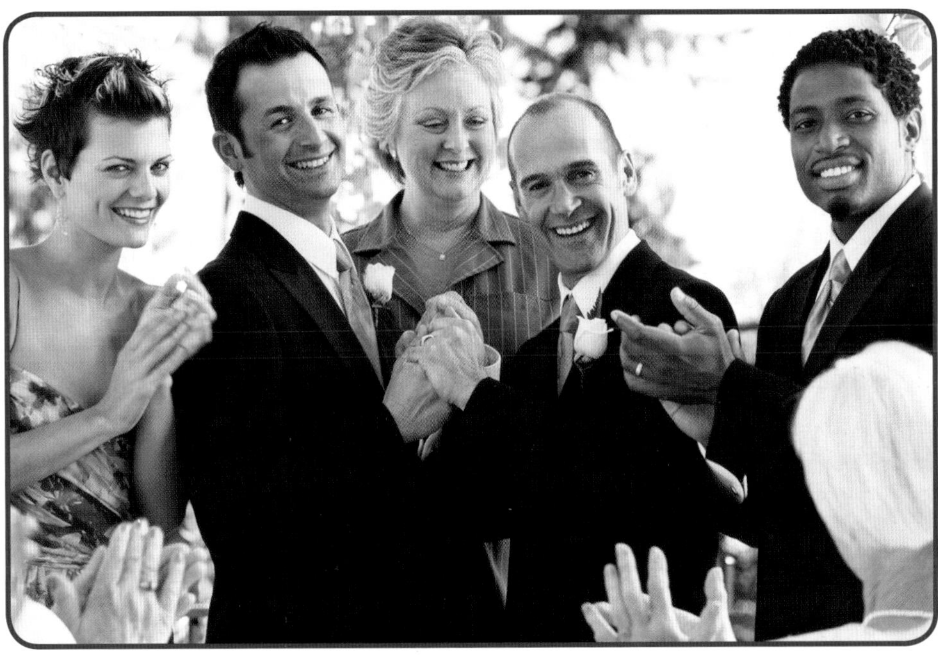

Figure 10.4 A wedding is an important life event

Task!

Think about different events or factors that have affected your physical health and experiences and your emotional and social well-being.

Assessment task 1.2 2.1

Using what you have learnt about Grace:

1 List three factors that may have affected her physical health and development during her lifetime.

2 List three experiences in Grace's life which may have affected her emotional and social well-being.

Summary

In this unit you have learned that:

- There are five main life stages.
- Factors such as diet, lifestyle and exercise can affect physical growth and development.
- Events such as the birth of a child or the death of a close family member are called 'life events'.
- Life events can affect a person's social and emotional well-being.

Chapter 11

Intro MU 1.7 Introduction to children and young people's development

What you will learn in this unit

- The stages of children and young people's development (0–19 years).
- The factors that affect children and young people's development.
- Ways to support children and young people's development.

Important words

Expected pattern of development – This is the order in which most people develop

Dependent – Needing the help and support of others

Independent – Not always needing the help and support of others

1.1 The expected pattern of development for children and young people (0–19 years)

During the time between birth and 19 years, a person will change from being dependent on their parents or carers who will have to meet all of their care needs, to becoming independent, able to look after themselves and manage their own lives.

There are four main areas of development; these are:

- physical development
- communication
- intellectual development
- social, emotional and behavioural development.

Expected patterns of development from birth to 12 months

Communication skills

At first a baby is only able to cry, but quickly learns to make cooing and gurgling sounds. During the first year of life a baby will begin to understand simple words such as their own name and the name of their pet.

Enjoys listening to songs and rhymes and by the age of 12 months knows and says one or two words and copies sounds.

Physical development

At birth a baby has reflexes such as sucking and grasping. A baby soon begins to control their body, for example using their hands to move objects or pull things towards them.

At around 8 months, a baby will begin to sit without support, and may start to crawl. Babies will begin to hold finger foods and drink from a trainer cup with handles from around 8 months.

Around 11 months a child may stand holding on to furniture or even take their first steps.

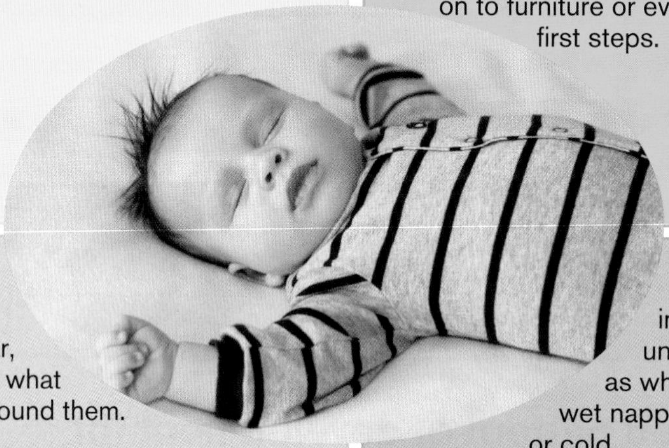

Intellectual development

A new baby begins to use senses to hear, smell and see what is going on around them.

From around 6 months, babies enjoy playing: moving toys and objects from one place to another so that by the time the baby is 12 months old, they are able to stack one brick on to another. Babies enjoy looking at bright colours.

Social and emotional development

A baby will cry when in pain, hungry or uncomfortable, such as when they have a wet nappy or feel too hot or cold.

By the age of 3 months, a baby may copy an adult's smile and will know the difference between family members.
A baby usually enjoys contact with family members, such as when feeding and being bathed.

At around 9 months, babies may become clingy with family members because they are now more aware of strangers.

Figure 11.1

Expected patterns of development from 12 months to 3 years

Communication skills

Children begin to repeat a few words around the age of 14 months and understand some instructions, such as 'coat on', 'come here'.

A child will put 3 or 4 words together to make sentences, for example, 'me do that' or 'little dog barking'.

Children will learn lots of new words and enjoy looking at picture books and listening to stories. By the age of 3 years, children will understand around 600 words.

Physical development

At 12 months children can usually stand without support and begin to walk. They begin to climb up stairs, so need to be watched! By the age of 2 years, a child can run, throw and kick a ball. By the time children are 3 years old, they have usually learned to jump off a low step and may ride a tricycle. They may also use a spoon and fork properly when feeding themselves.

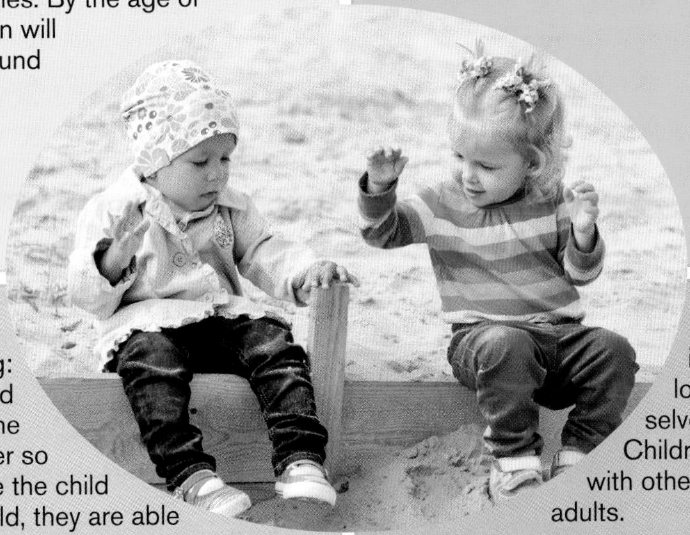

Intellectual development

Children begin to enjoy playing: moving toys and objects from one place to another so that by the time the child is 18 months old, they are able to stack three or four bricks in a tower.

Children may enjoy play dough and messy activities. As children get older they may enjoy listening to others count and may begin to join in. They may also enjoy listening to stories and know the names of the characters in their favourite stories.

Social and emotional development

A child may be interested in looking at themselves in the mirror. Children enjoy playing with other children and adults.

Understand the meaning of different facial expressions; for example, children will know when a person is happy or sad.

Figure 11.2

Expected patterns of development from 3–5 years

Communication skills

By 4 years children can understand over 1,000 words and make sentences of 5 or more words.

Children now enjoy listening to longer stories and will often choose the same story over and over again.

Children at 5 years know up to 2,000 words and use proper sentences. Children often talk clearly and will enjoy telling stories about themselves.

Physical development

Stands on one leg, jumps up and down.

Enjoys climbing and can change direction quickly when running in the play area.

May now be able to take responsibility for their own toileting. Can open and close fastening; can dress and undress for a PE lesson.

Can use scissors to cut out shapes and pictures. Skips with a rope. Runs quickly and safely around the playground without bumping into other children.

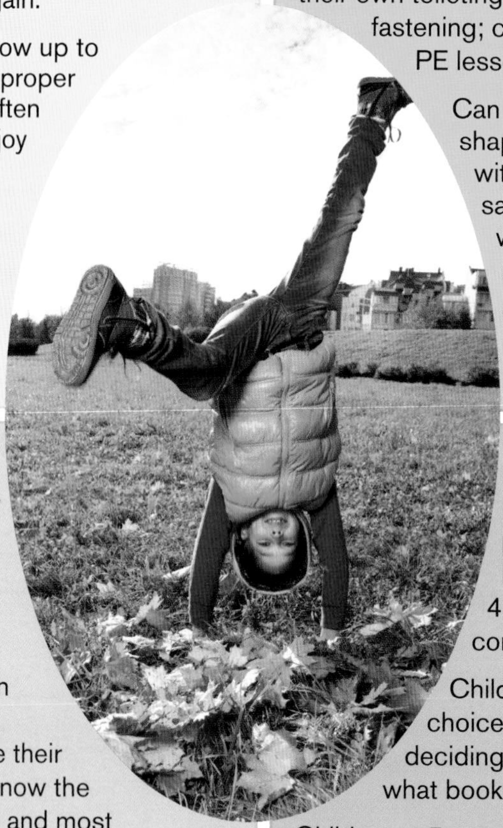

Intellectual development

By the age of 3 years children begin to enjoy counting up to ten and begin to learn the names of colours and shapes.

At the age of 4 children may copy letters and numbers and may write their own name. They may know the names of most colours and most simple shapes.

At the age of 5 years children may draw pictures of trees, houses, people and animals. Can complete a 20-piece jigsaw puzzle.

Social and emotional development

Likes to spend time playing alone but also enjoys playing with other children. Enjoys caring for pets. At 4 years children show concern when a friend is hurt.

Children will like to make choices for themselves, such as deciding which clothes to wear or what book to look at.

Children at 5 years usually enjoy being busy and playing co-operatively. This means that they can agree rules of a game and take turns.

Figure 11.3

Expected patterns of development from 5–11 years

Communication skills

During this time children become more and more independent and will possibly spend less time with their families as they get older, as they want to spend time with friends.

Children can agree rules during play and will give and take instructions.

Children can read the body language of other people and can understand how someone feels by their tone of voice.

Physical development

At this age children's balance and co-ordination improve. Children can become very skilled in an activity or sport, such as ballet or football.

Up to the age of 11 years children will be able to gain more difficult skills using their hands, such as knitting, model making and building with small bricks.

Children will begin to be able to care for themselves physically, such as washing own hair and cleaning their teeth.

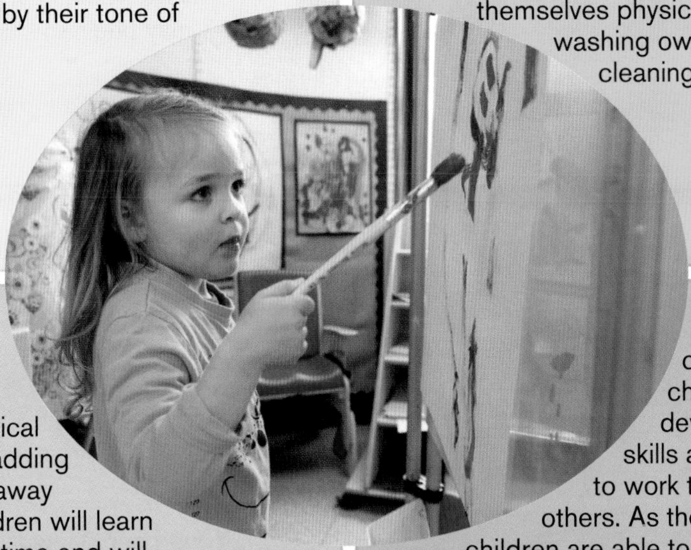

Intellectual development

Children at primary school will be developing mathematical skills such as adding up and taking away numbers. Children will learn how to tell the time and will understand about seasons and changes in the weather.

Older children will be able to do more complicated maths problems and will be developing a good understanding of the world around them.

Social and emotional development

Between the ages of 5 and 11 years, children are developing social skills and learning how to work together with others. As they get older, children are able to see things from the other person's point of view when having a discussion.

Children at this age are very aware of social rules and how to behave; they will understand what may happen when they break any rules.

Figure 11.4

Expected patterns of development from 11–19 years

Communication skills

Young people will use their communication skills to put across their own views and opinions. Some young people at this age find it more and more difficult to communicate with parents and adults in authority, such as teachers, often finding it easier to communicate with others who are their own age.

Physical development

There are many physical changes taking place during this stage, which is known as adolescence. Bodies go through changes linked to reproduction. Hormones affect growth of bones and muscles, mood and appearance, such as hair growth.

Girls will develop breasts and their periods will begin during this stage.

Boys' voices deepen and they may begin to shave.

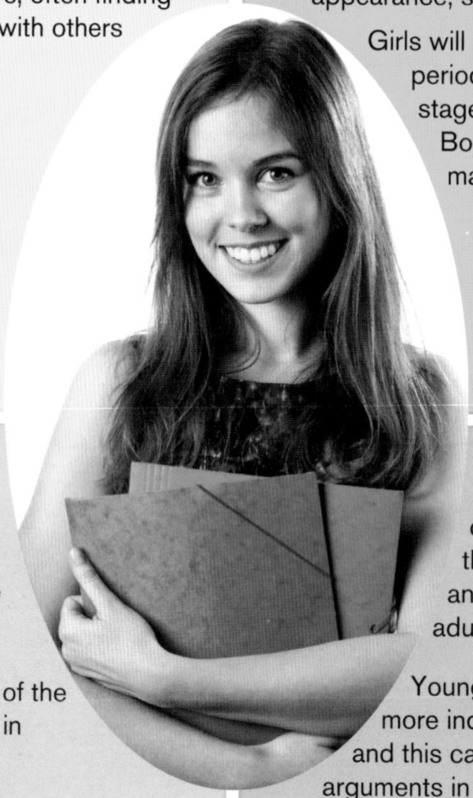

Intellectual development

Young people are very aware of the world around them and understand how things work. Many young people are skilled at using the computer or are very interested in one or more of the subjects they learn about in school.

Young people will often start to take an interest in the wider wold, such as listening to world news or what is happening in their local area.

Social and emotional development

Some adolescents find this time can be emotionally difficult as they get used to the changes in their bodies and they become more like adults.

Young people usually want to be more independent during this stage and this can sometimes cause arguments in families.

During this time, girls and boys may have relationships which can be special to them but may also cause problems for them emotionally.

Figure 11.5

Assessment task 1.1

Design a wall display which shows the expected pattern of development for children and young people 0–19 years. Include:

- physical development
- communication
- intellectual development
- social and emotional development.

2.1 Factors that affect children and young people's development

There are a number of factors that can affect children's growth and development

Background

A child or young person's background including their personal history (this is what has happened in their lives so far), such as loss of a parent or unhealthy lifestyle choices, affects their development. Culture and religious beliefs may also affect social development, as some children and young people are expected only to mix in their own groups.

Language development is mostly affected by the way that children are spoken to and communicated with when they are young. If a child is encouraged to talk and is included in conversations, for example asking the child what they did when they went to nursery or asking them about pictures in a book, it will support their language development. Children copy what they hear, so it is very important for young people and adults to only use appropriate language around a young child. If a child hears others using swear words, or they hear people around them saying unkind things, the child will copy this and they might use this language when they are at school, which could get them into trouble, which may upset the child. Adults should be good role models for young children, especially when working in health and social care and childcare.

Family relationships

The family can have a big effect on a child or young person's development. If the child spends time with members of their family, playing games, reading stories or going out to places, their development will be supported. For example if a child goes shopping with family members they will be seeing the world around them and learning new things; they might also see how to communicate well. If parents or carers are responsible carers, giving time to their children and showing them care and kindness, this can support children's development. If however a child or young person does not have the chance to spend good quality time with family members they may not understand about good trusting relationships, they may not have their care needs met and they may not feel secure and this can affect their development.

Health

Health can be affected by the choices a person makes, by the environment or by their physical health and can include:

Diet

A good, well-balanced diet will help to support children's healthy growth and development.

A poor diet might mean that children and young people are not getting all the vitamins and nutrients they need to keep their bodies healthy. They may also have too much salt, fat or sugar in their diet which could cause health problems.

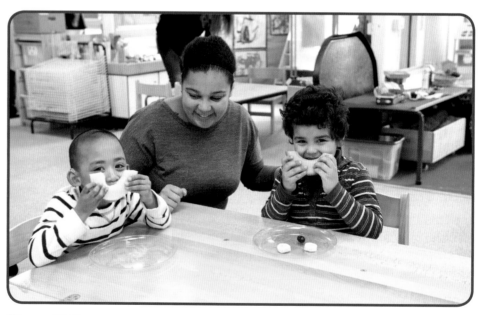

Figure 11.6

Exercise

Exercise gives children and young people the chance to use their muscles to become strong, flexible and healthy.

Not enough exercise might cause muscles to become weak. They may build up too much body fat and become ill later in life.

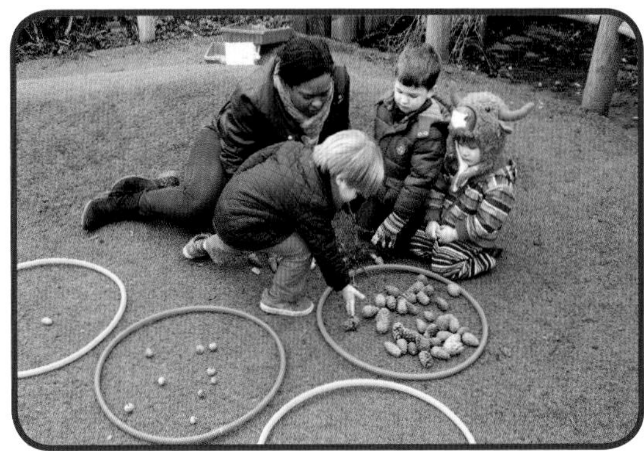

Figure 11.7

Illness

Illness can affect growth and development. Some illnesses can mean that a child may stop growing or grows very slowly.

Illness affects a child or young person's development as they may spend time in hospital or be unable to go to school to learn and to meet with their friends. They may not be able to develop intellectually (learn new things) or develop good social skills.

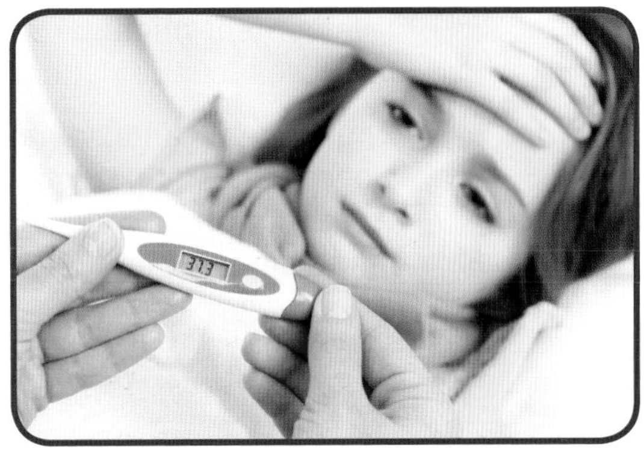

Figure 11.8

Disability

Disability may affect a child or young person's development if they are not given the correct support from adults. For example, a child who needs glasses might not be able to see pictures in a book or the computer screen clearly.

However, if a young person using a wheelchair is given the correct support, he or she should be able to enjoy most activities with others.

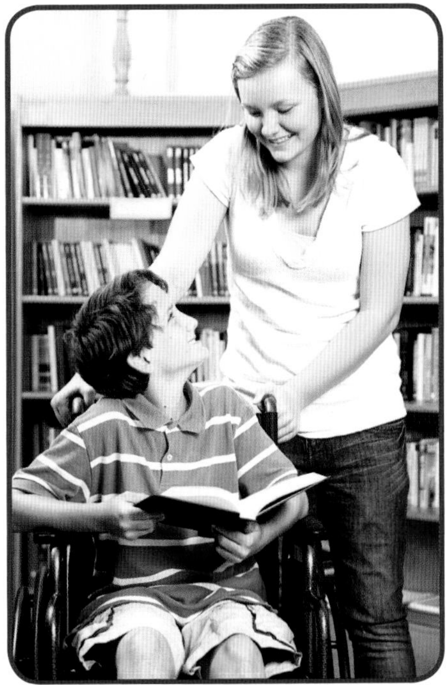

Figure 11.9

Environment

The environment or the world around a child or young person can affect their development, for example:

The lifestyle of the family can have a good or bad effect on the child or young person's development. If adults smoke in the house, close to where the child or young person is sleeping or playing, they could have some breathing difficulties and hearing problems known as 'glue ear'.

The amount of money a family has can affect a child or young person; for example if there is not enough money to buy warm clothes or to go on trips and visits the child's development might be affected.

If the child has lots of space to run and play outdoors they will have more opportunities to develop physically; however, if they live in an area where it is not very safe to play outdoors, for example they live beside a busy road or in a tall block of flats, they might not have the chance to play outdoors so often.

A young person might live next to noisy neighbours and might not get a good amount of sleep each night, so their intellectual development may be affected if they cannot concentrate at school. If the house is crowded there might not be a quiet place to do homework, so again intellectual development might be affected compared to a young person who has a quite area to study at home.

Employment can also have an effect on a child's development. This is because if the parents work it might mean the child goes to a day nursery or other childcare and the quality of this care will affect the child's development.

Assessment task 2.1

Make a poster showing the different factors that can affect children's growth and development, including:

- background
- health
- environment.

3.1 Outline different ways to support children and young people's development

Children and young people need help and support to develop and there are many ways that this help and support can be given. Some ways include:

- physical development
- social, emotional and behavioural development.
- communication
- intellectual development

Task!

Using what you have read in this chapter so far, complete the circle diagrams to suggest ways to support children and young people's development.

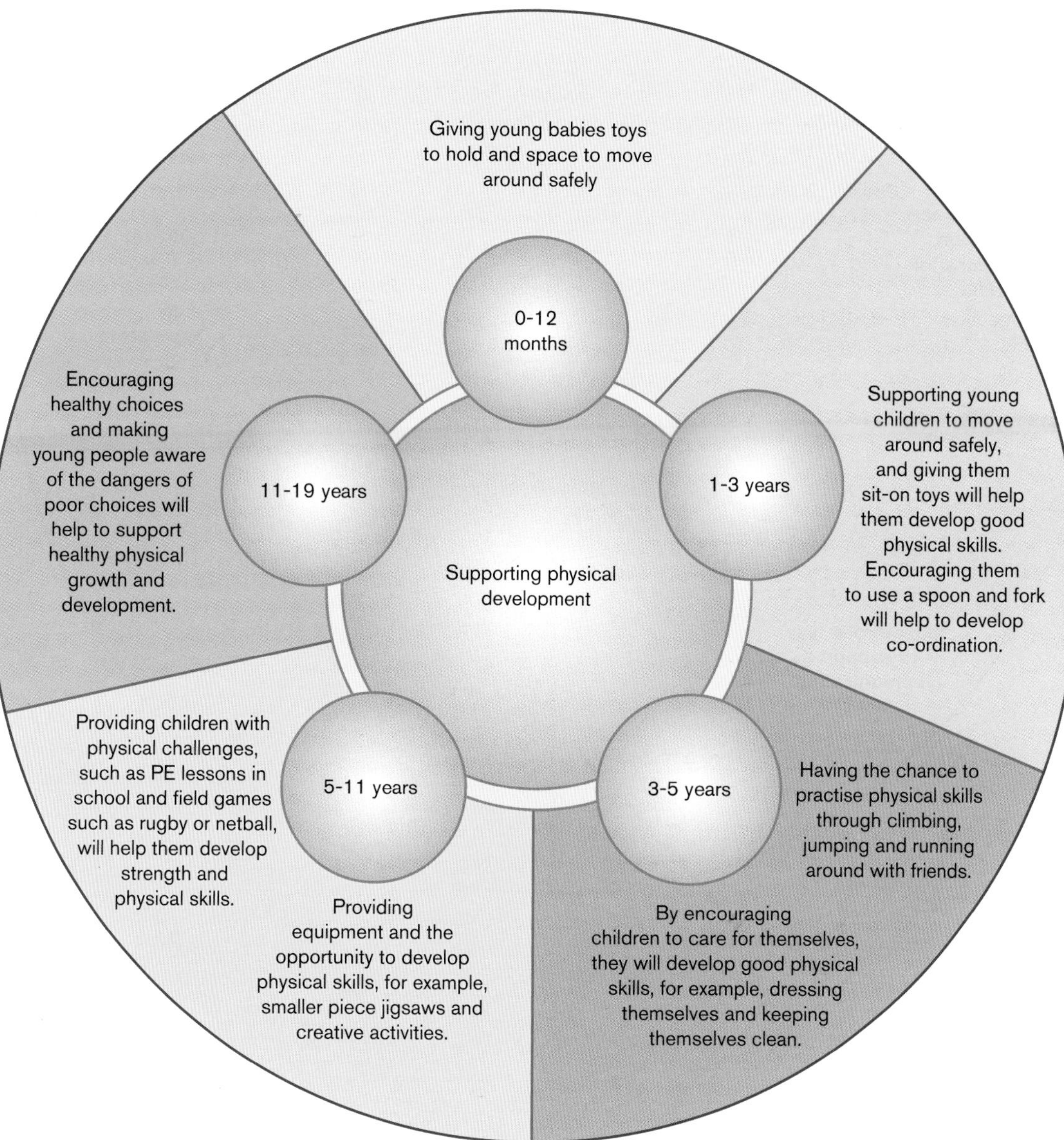

Figure 11.10 Supporting physical development

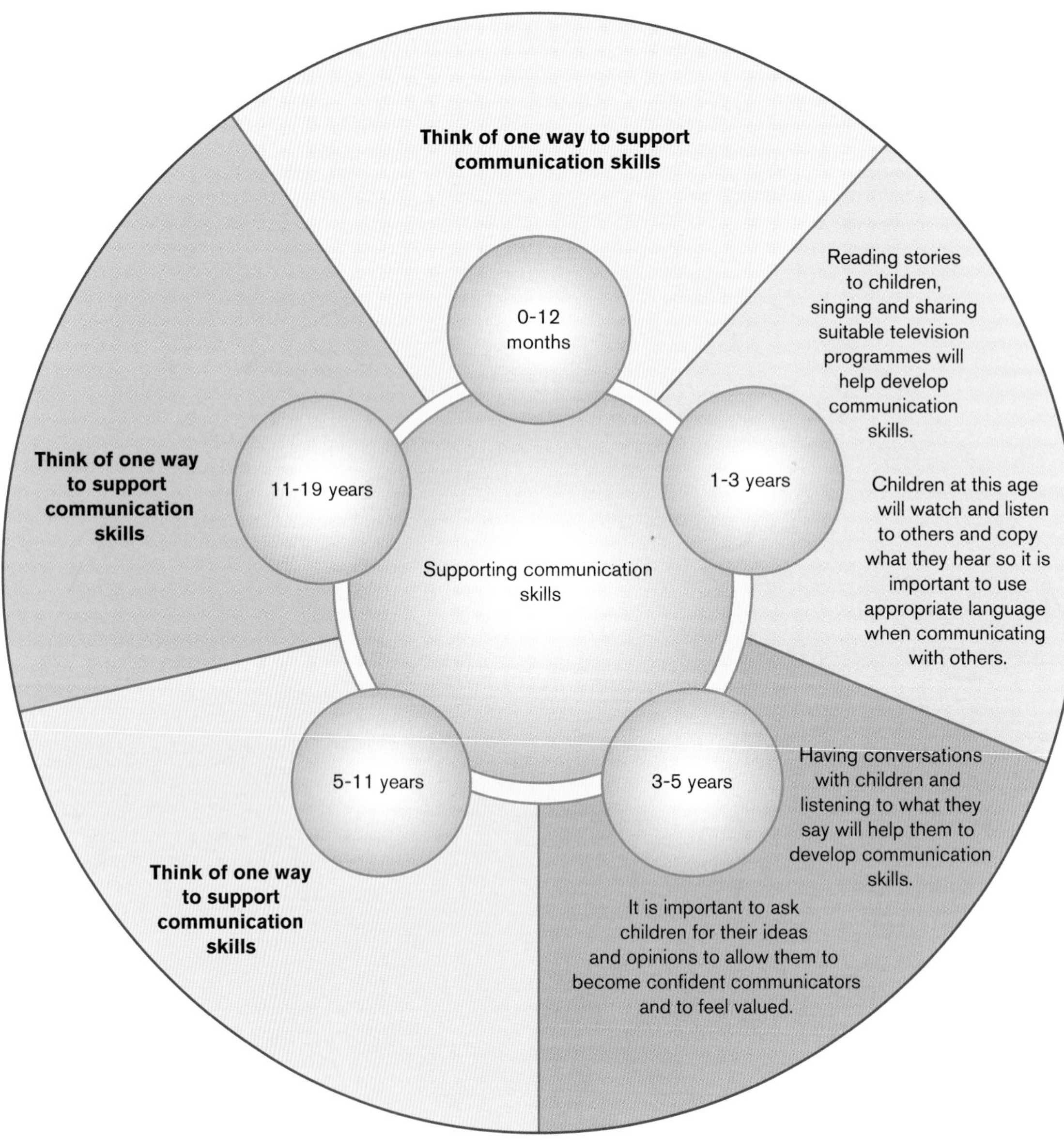

Figure 11.11 Supporting communication skills

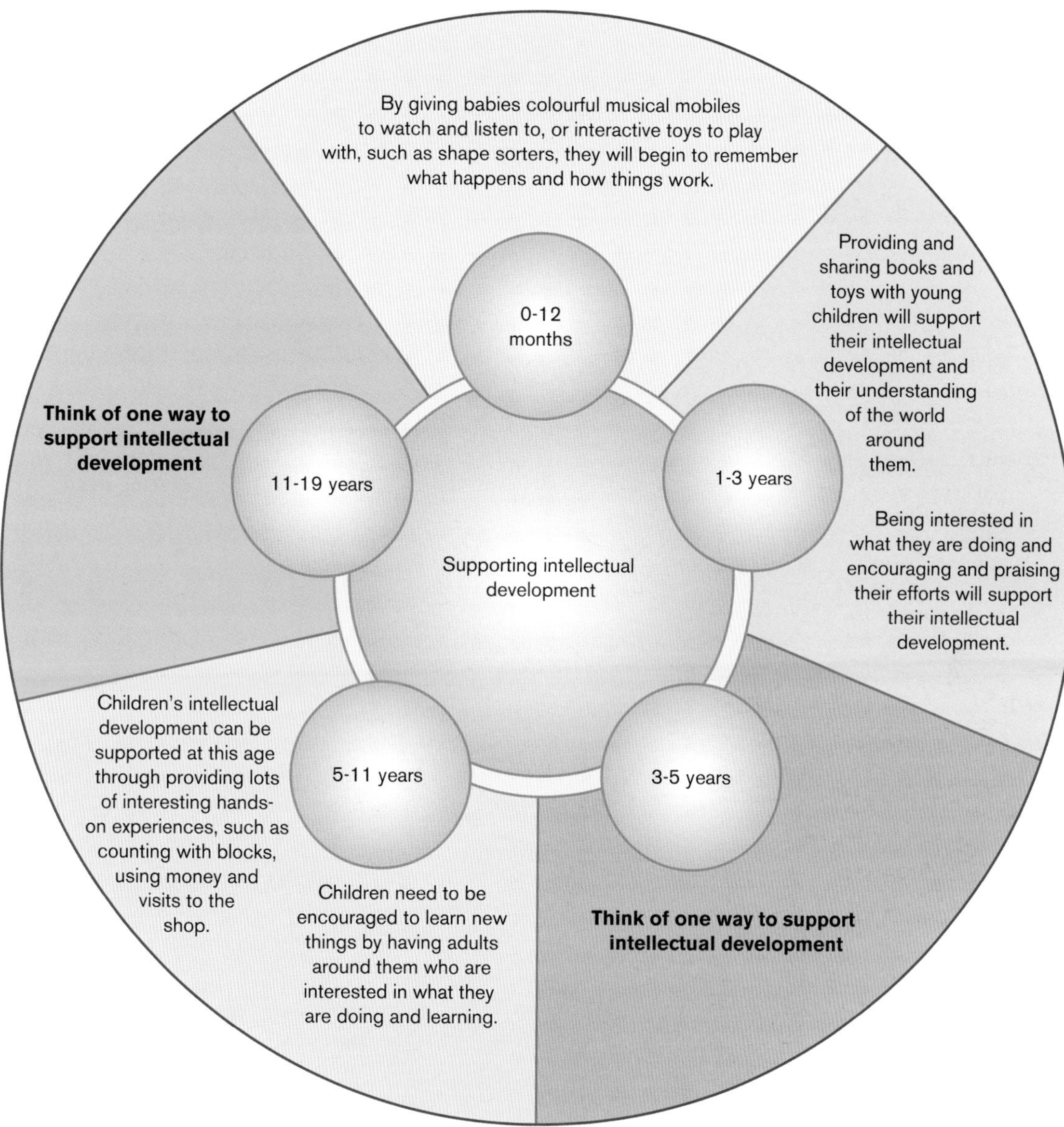

By giving babies colourful musical mobiles to watch and listen to, or interactive toys to play with, such as shape sorters, they will begin to remember what happens and how things work.
0-12 months
Providing and sharing books and toys with young children will support their intellectual development and their understanding of the world around them.
1-3 years
Being interested in what they are doing and encouraging and praising their efforts will support their intellectual development.
3-5 years
Think of one way to support intellectual development
Children need to be encouraged to learn new things by having adults around them who are interested in what they are doing and learning.
5-11 years
Children's intellectual development can be supported at this age through providing lots of interesting hands-on experiences, such as counting with blocks, using money and visits to the shop.
11-19 years
Think of one way to support intellectual development
Supporting intellectual development

Figure 11.12 Supporting intellectual development

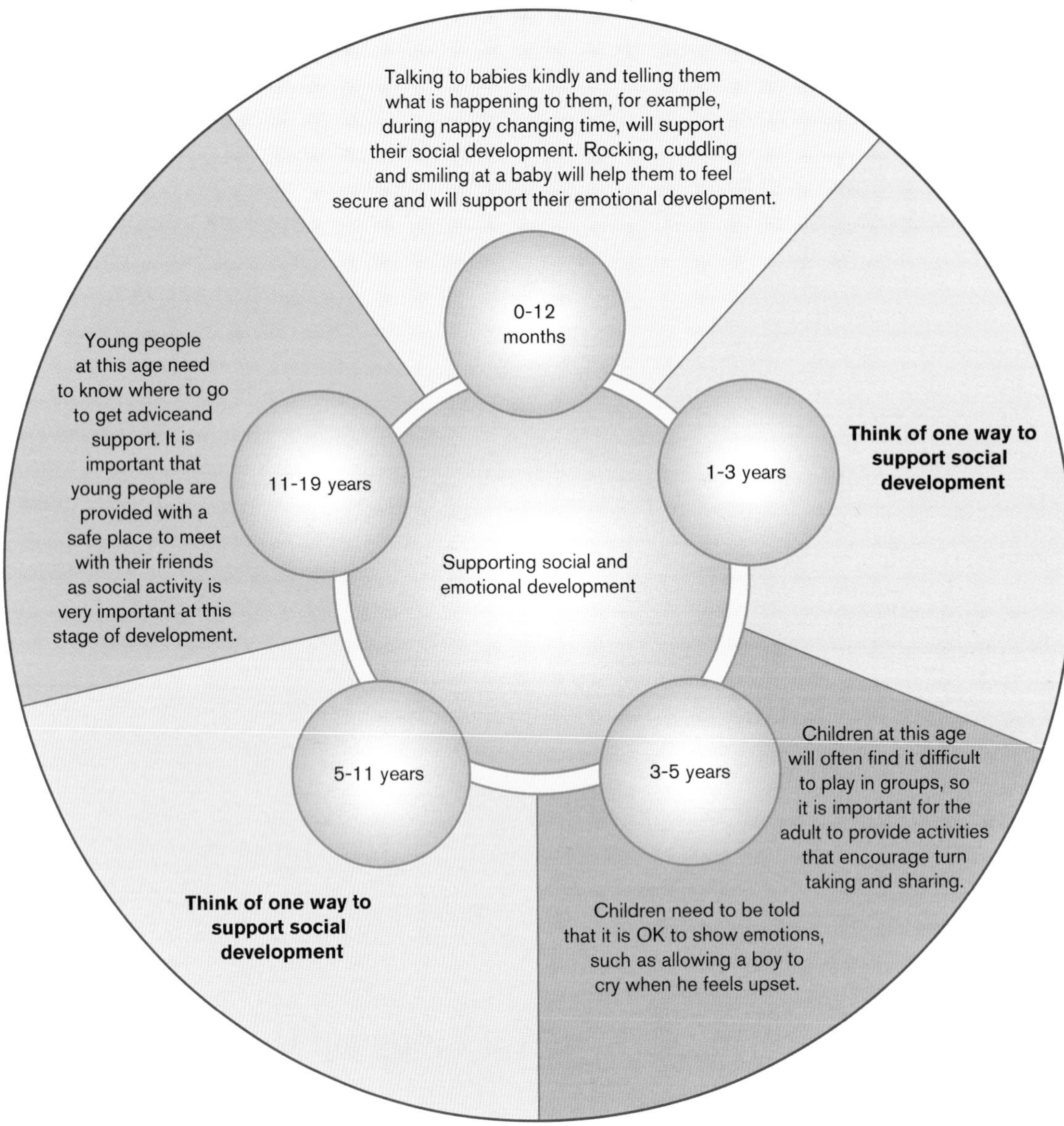

Figure 11.13 Supporting social and emotional development

Assessment task 3.1

Adding to the wall display, include information to show the different ways to show children and young people's development. Include a minimum of two examples for each of the following areas:

- physical development
- communication
- intellectual development
- social, emotional and behavioural development.

Summary

In this unit you have learned that:

- Children and young people 0–19 years go through several main stages of development.
- There are many factors that affect children and young people's development.
- There are good ways to support children and young people's development.

Chapter 12

Intro Op 1.1 Understand the importance of engagement in leisure and social activities in health and social care

What you will learn in this unit

- The importance of leisure and social activities for an individual's well-being.
- How leisure and social activities support relationships.
- A range of leisure and social activities.
- How to find out about the interests and preferences of individuals.
- The benefits of a person-centred approach for individuals taking part in leisure or social activities.
- The different types of support that individuals may need to take part in leisure and social activities.
- How to promote independence through leisure and social activities.

Important words

Leisure activities – Interests or hobbies that people can enjoy

Social activities – Free time that people can enjoy with others

Well-being – Health and happiness

Support relationships – spending time with others to strengthen friendships and meet new people

1.1 1.2 Outline why leisure and social activities are important for an individual's well-being and support relationships

Everybody needs to spend time relaxing and doing the things that they enjoy, either on their own or with friends. Leisure activities give children and adults the chance to take part in activities that will interest them and help them to relax. For example, children may enjoy riding their bike in the local park and older adults may enjoy walking in the countryside. These sorts of activities are very important for an **individual's well-being** because they help people to keep fit and healthy and also boost happiness, helping them to feel less stressed or unhappy.

Children and adults may spend time enjoying leisure activities with other individuals or groups. For example, a child may visit the local park with friends from school and an older aged adult may belong to a walking club which meets every weekend to walk together as a group. Taking part in social activities or hobbies helps to **support relationships** because people have the chance to make new friends and also to enjoy friendships with people that they already know. Family leisure activities also allow families to strengthen their relationships and spend quality time together.

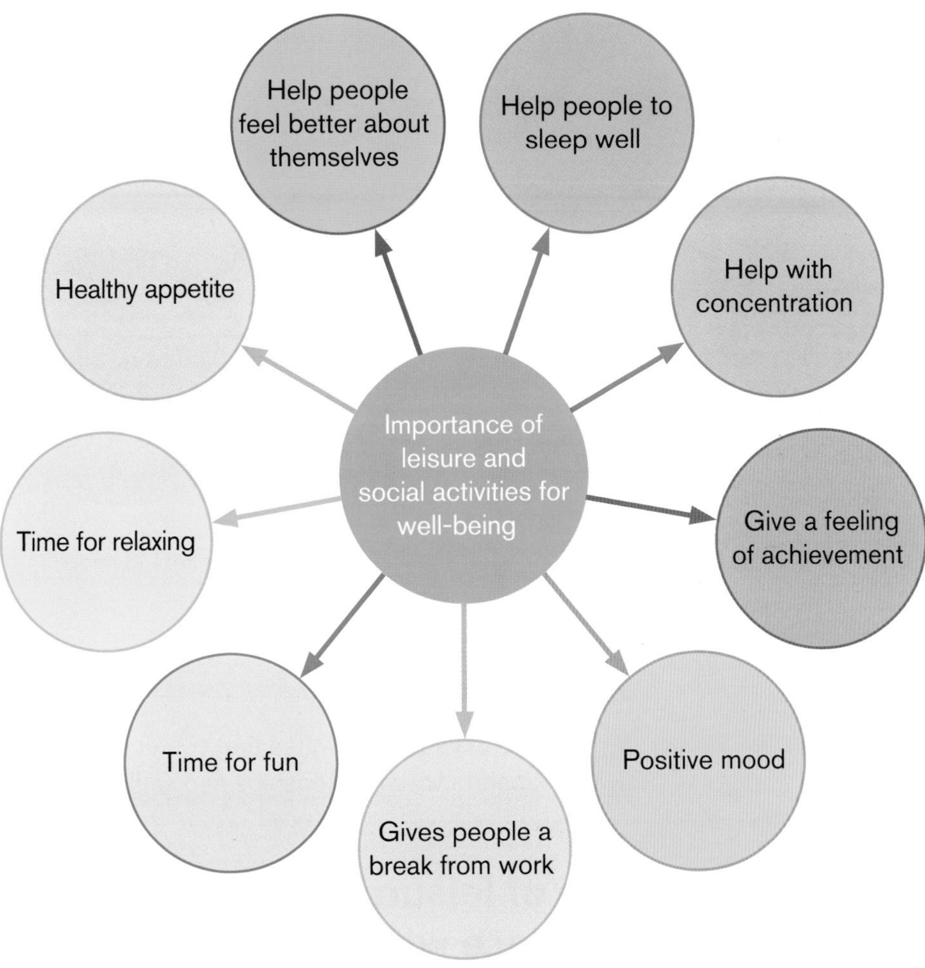

Figure 12.1 Importance of leisure and social activities for well-being

Give feeling of belonging
People can support each other
Help people feel more confident

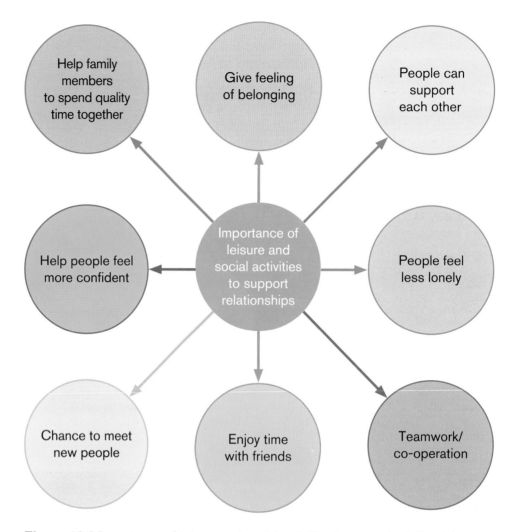

People feel less lonely

Teamwork/ co-operation

Figure 12.2 Importance of leisure and social activities to support relationships

Assessment task 1.1 1.2

Make a poster showing the leisure and social activities that you enjoy and say how doing these activities supports your relationships and well-being.

2.1 Identify a range of leisure and social activities that take place within:

- a person's own home
- a local community
- a residential or group living home
- day care provision.

There are many different leisure and social activities that can be enjoyed by children and adults, either in their own home, in different health and social care settings or within the local community.

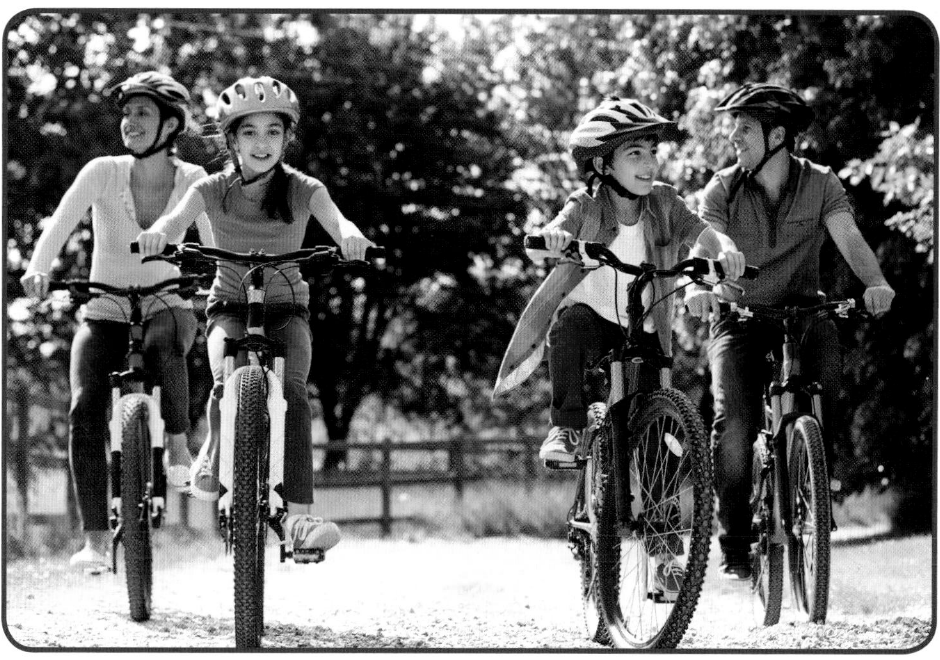

Figure 12.3 A family enjoying a bike trip

Place of leisure or social activity	Leisure or social activity			
A person's home	Dinner party with friends	Reading a book or watching a film	Coffee mornings	Gardening
A local community	Tennis club	Singing in the local choir	Swimming club	Craft fair
A residential or group living home	Playing bingo	Group trip to the coast	Watching old films	Visit from family and friends
Day care provision	Sewing and knitting groups	Flower arranging	Sing-a-longs	Lunch clubs

Table 12.1 Different social and leisure activities and where they can take place

Assessment task 2.1

Make your own table like the one above to show different leisure and social activities that can take place in:

- a local community
- a person's own home
- a residential home
- day care provision.

3.1 How to find out about the interests and preferences of individuals

There are many ways to find out about the interests and preferences of individuals and these include:

- asking a person about their interests
- giving a person choices
- using questionnaires or suggestion boxes
- talking to families and carers
- observing their reactions to things
- looking at personal records
- providing a range of leisure and social activities.

Assessment task 3.1

John is 20 years old and has learning difficulties. He will be attending a day care centre for two days each week.

How can the carers working in the centre find out about John's interests and preferences?

3.2 The benefits for individuals of a person-centred approach when taking part in leisure or social activities

Taking the person-centred approach will make it easier to provide leisure and social activities that a person enjoys. This is because the interests and preferences of individuals come first.

This is different to not having a person-centred approach. For example, in a care home a few activities may be provided by the care workers, even if the residents are not very interested in that type of activity.

Listening to a person to find out about their interests, likes and dislikes and using this information to provide suitable activities means that a person-centred approach is being used.

By taking a person-centred approach when planning activities, carers will be able to make sure that the activity is safe for the individual.

There are many benefits to using a person-centred approach when providing leisure and social activities. These may include:

- A person will want to take part in the activity.
- A person may do well in the activity if it is something that they enjoy.
- The person may feel good about themselves if they do well in the activity.
- The person might make friends with others who enjoy the same activity.
- The person might have fun and feel happy.
- The person may have skills to share with others.
- The person's own skills might improve.
- The activity will be safe for the individual

Assessment task 3.2

John is now settled into the day care centre and is taking part in the activities. The carers have used a person-centred approach to provide the activities. How will John benefit from this?

3.3 The different types of support that individuals may need to take part in leisure and social activities

There are many types of support that may be needed when individuals take part in leisure or social activities. It may be that an individual needs help to get somewhere such as to a community or sports centre to take part in an activity. This support could mean someone drives them to the centre or perhaps walks with them if it is close by.

When the person is at the community or sports centre, they may have the support of an instructor or group leader and may also get support from others taking part in the activity.

When a person is less able to do things for themselves, they may need a care worker to set out the activity or to support them to take part. For example, if individuals in a residential home for older aged adults are enjoying a dancing session, a person in a wheelchair may enjoy being pushed around the dance floor by a carer so they can join in.

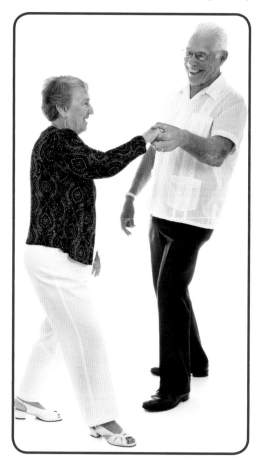

Figure 12.4

Assessment task 3.3

Describe the different types of support that individuals may need to take part in leisure and social activities within:

- the community
- their own home
- a residential home.

3.4 How to promote independence through leisure and social activities

It is important that care workers allow individuals to be as independent as possible because if they start doing everything for a person, that person may lose their skills, or stop trying to do things for themselves. To promote independence through activities, it is important to:

- Let a person choose their own activities.
- Only give support that a person asks for.
- Let a person know you are there to help when needed.
- Take an interest and join in, without taking over.
- Take notice and praise a person when they do well or try hard.

Assessment task 3.4

Read the list above and, in small groups, make a list of other ways to promote independence through leisure and social activities.

Summary

In this unit you have learned:

- the importance of leisure and social activities for an individual's well-being
- how leisure and social activities support relationships
- that there are many leisure and social activities
- how to find out about the interests and preferences of individuals
- the benefits of a person-centred approach for individuals taking part in leisure or social activities
- the different types of support that individuals may need to take part in leisure and social activities
- how to promote independence through leisure and social activities.

Chapter 13

Intro Op 1.2 Introduction to a healthy lifestyle

What you will learn in this unit

- What contributes to a healthy lifestyle.
- How activities contribute to a healthy lifestyle.
- What contributes to an unhealthy lifestyle.
- The positive and negative parts of own lifestyle.
- Developing a personal healthy lifestyle plan.

Important words

Contributes – Helps to support
Lifestyle – Way of life
Releases – Frees
Hinder – Stop

1.1 Factors that contribute to a healthy lifestyle

The main factors that contribute to a healthy lifestyle include:

- diet
- exercise
- work and play
- rest and sleep.

1.2 Benefits of living a healthy lifestyle

Diet

The food and drinks that we take into our bodies have an effect on our health. This means it is important to eat a wide variety of foods in the right amounts to have a healthy body weight. We must also drink lots of fluids to keep our bodies hydrated. We need to eat a good balanced diet that contains all the nutrients needed for growth and good health.

Eating too much food or having a poor diet, such as eating lots of takeaway food which is high in fat and salt or having too many sugary drinks, can make us overweight. Not eating enough good foods such as fruit, vegetables and whole grains can leave us feeling tired and our bodies may not be able to fight off illness.

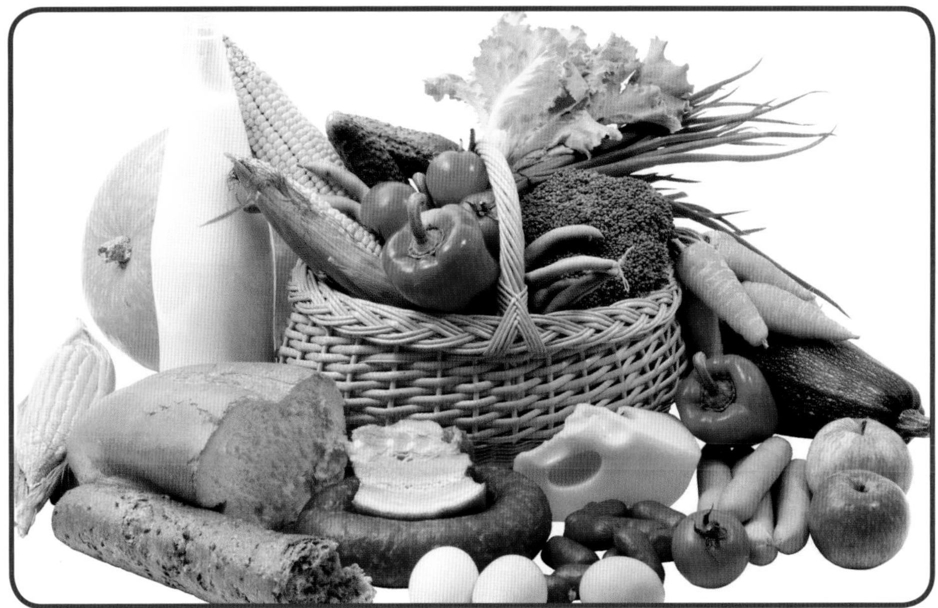

Figure 13.1 Healthy foods

Exercise

Regular exercise plays an important part in keeping us healthy; this is because when we exercise we use energy to burn calories and body fat, and muscles become toned and strong.

Regular exercise can help us to relax and sleep well. It also helps to fight disease such as heart disease and high blood pressure. Exercise, as well as being fun, also releases chemicals in our bodies that help to put us into a good mood and help us to relax.

Work and play

Work and play can both benefit a healthy lifestyle. For example if a person works regularly they will need to be in a routine where they get out of bed and get ready for work. When working, people will be using their skills and perhaps learning new skills. The type of work a person does might mean that they have to work as part of a team or perhaps make decisions for themselves; this may help to develop confidence or improve communication skills. Both work and play can make a person feel proud that they have achieved something or completed a task well.

When a person is out of work they may feel bored or their self-esteem may suffer.

Rest and sleep

Sleep is important for us because this is the time when bodies grow and repair themselves; sleep allows us to fight off infection and disease. When we sleep, we store memories and make sense of the world around us.

When we have had enough sleep we are able to concentrate for longer and remember things more clearly. A good night's sleep leaves us feeling fresh and full of energy, ready for the day ahead.

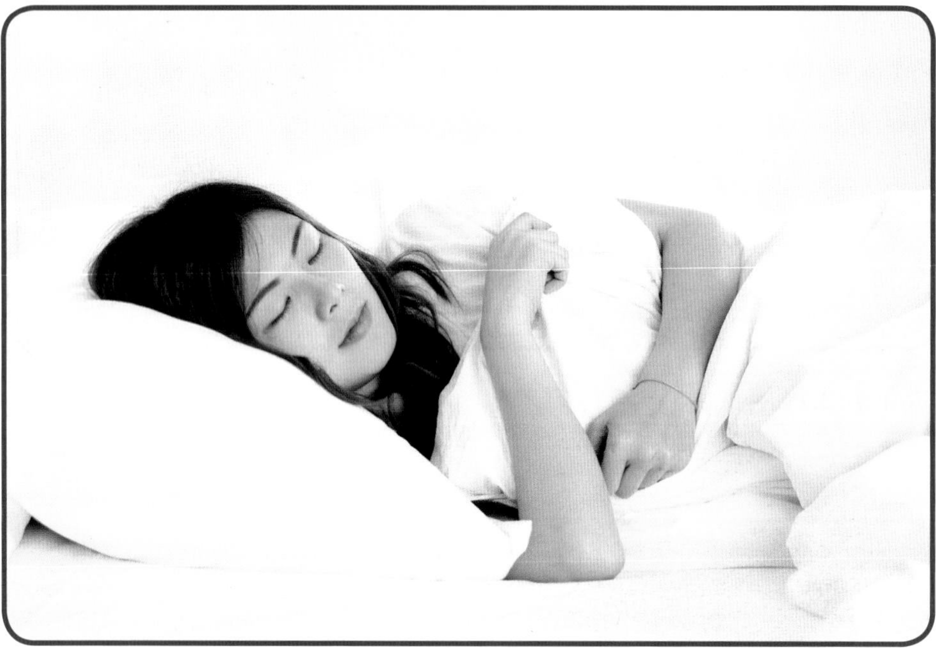

Figure 13.2 A good night's sleep leaves us feeling fresh and full of energy

Assessment task 1.1 1.2

Write a page for a health magazine to give information about healthy lifestyles, including:

- the factors that contribute to a healthy lifestyle
- the benefits of a healthy lifestyle.

2.1 Activities in the local area that support a healthy lifestyle

Activities in your local area may include:

- swimming
- football
- yoga
- tennis
- basketball
- netball
- bowling
- aerobics classes
- dance classes
- judo
- walking and running.

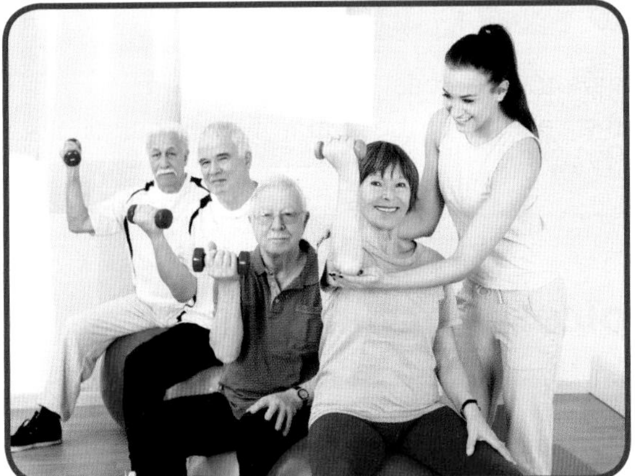

Figure 13.3

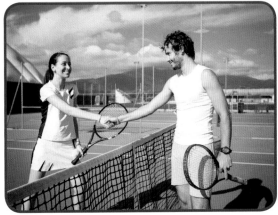

Figure 13.4

2.2 2.3 The benefits of selected activities on personal well-being as a result of taking part in activities

There are many benefits of taking part in activities that support a healthy lifestyle. The benefits can be physical, such as strengthening muscles and fighting infection, and emotional, such as enjoying spending time with friends or feeling good about doing well in the activity.

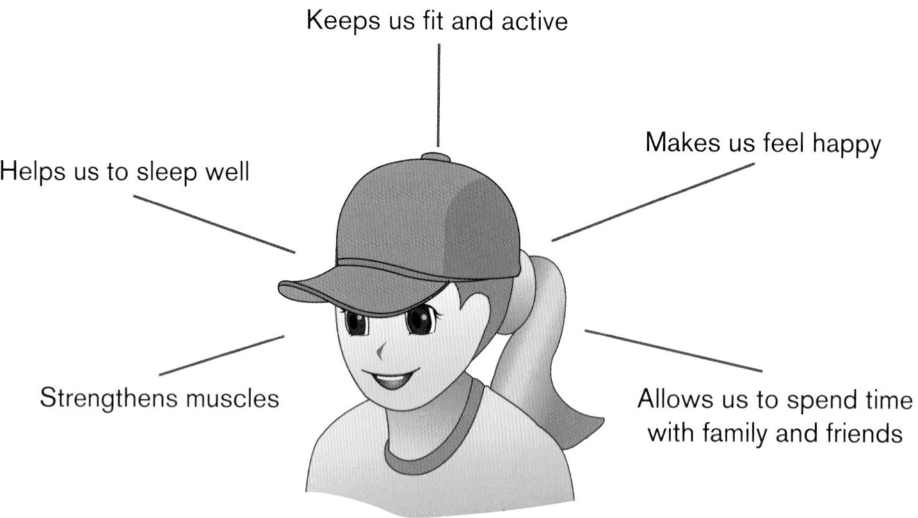
Keeps us fit and active
Makes us feel happy
Helps us to sleep well
Strengthens muscles
Allows us to spend time with family and friends

Figure 13.5 The benefits of taking part in activities that support a healthy lifestyle

Assessment task 2.1 2.2 2.3

On your page for the health magazine list at least three activities in your local area and write about the benefits of these activities on personal well-being.

3.1 Activities and choices that hinder a healthy lifestyle

There are a few activities and choices that stop us from having a healthy lifestyle and we should try to avoid these as much as we can.

Activities and choices to avoid include:

- smoking
- using drugs and alcohol
- eating a poor diet
- lack of exercise
- lack of sleep.

3.2 How these activities and choices can have a negative effect on personal well-being

There are many ways that making poor choices and leading an unhealthy lifestyle can have a negative effect on personal well-being. Eating an unhealthy diet or not exercising enough may mean that we develop too much body fat, feel tired or become unwell. Lack of sleep may make us feel irritable or unable to concentrate properly.

Smoking, drinking too much alcohol and using drugs all damage our body and can cause illness and disease.

Assessment task 3.1 3.2

On your health magazine page:

- List at least three choices that can stop a person from having a healthy lifestyle.
- Say how these choices negatively affect the body.

4.1 Identifying positive and negative aspects of your own lifestyle

We all make choices about our lifestyle and these choices affect our physical and emotional well-being. For example, if we eat too many takeaway meals, we could be eating too much sugar and salt and not getting the right nutrients to keep us healthy.

Each day we make choices that affect our physical and emotional well-being without thinking about it. For example, we may take the lift instead of using the stairs or choose water instead of a sugary drink. All of these choices will have an effect on our health and well-being.

4.2 Produce an action plan to improve own health and well-being

It is important that we all try to have a healthy lifestyle. This means that we sometimes have to make changes in the choices we usually make.

Assessment task 4.1 4.2

Complete the table below to show the positive and negative aspects of your own lifestyle and show ways to make healthy changes.

Positive and negative aspects of my lifestyle	Activities and choices that will improve my health and well-being
I drink a bit too much alcohol on Fridays and Saturdays	I will choose more non-alcoholic drinks I will try to only drink two glasses of beer when I go out on Friday and Saturday nights
I always walk the dog in the park after dinner	I will continue to take the dog for a walk because I know this exercise is helping me to stay healthy

Summary

In this unit you have learned that:

- Some activities and choices help us to have a healthy lifestyle.
- Some activities and choices mean we have an unhealthy lifestyle.
- We can look at the positive and negative aspects of our own lifestyles and make a plan to help us get fitter and healthier.

Chapter 14

Intro Op 1.6 Introduction to physical disability

What you will learn in this unit

- The importance of recognising and valuing children, young people and adults with a physical disability.
- The main causes of physical disability.
- The challenges of living with a physical disability.

Important words

Discriminatory attitudes – The poor attitude and behaviour people show towards others with disability

Promoting independence – Encouraging someone to find ways to do things for themselves

Inclusion – Being part of something, being included, or making sure everyone can be included

1.1 The importance of recognising and valuing individuals with a physical disability

It is very important to see an individual with physical disability as a person with feelings and needs first, rather than focusing on the disability first.

It is important to value the person first for many reasons. One reason is that there is a law called the 'Equality Act 2012' which says that any person with a disability must have the same opportunities as those without a disability. This means that it is against the law for anyone to discriminate against someone with a disability.

It is important to understand what support a person with a disability might need to live their daily lives as normally as possible. It is important that a person with a disability has the same opportunities in life as people without a disability; this is called 'having equal opportunities'. In order to give people with disability equal opportunities, special equipment is sometimes needed or help and support from other people may be needed.

Equal opportunity does not mean treating everyone the same; it means looking at individual needs and finding ways to give everyone a chance to take part. For example, not everyone with a physical disability requires a wheelchair, so just having wheelchairs available will not suit all people with a disability.

People with a physical disability should be allowed to make as many decisions as they can for themselves so that they feel in control of their own lives. By valuing the person, and not seeing the disability first, the needs of the person can be more easily understood. By valuing the person with a physical disability, the person will know that their opinions and feelings matter and they may feel more able to make important decisions about what happens to them and this may help them to feel more in control of their own lives.

1.2 Examples of using the person-centred approach when working with individuals with a physical disability

To use the person-centred approach, care workers or health professionals should have a good understanding of the needs of the person with a disability. Care workers should take time to find out about the person's opinions, needs, likes and dislikes by asking the right questions and listening carefully to their answers.

The person-centred approach makes sure the person with a disability is listened to and their opinions are valued. It may be that the person with a disability likes to do things in a different way to others and the person-centred approach allows the person to make their own choices. Care workers using the person-centred approach should give people with disability every chance to be able to make choices for themselves.

Often people with a physical disability feel that they struggle to do the things that able-bodied people can easily do and they can feel very frustrated and upset. The person-centred approach means that care workers need to show they understand the difficulties that the person with a physical disability might have and be able to offer the right choices of support.

Assessment task 1.1 1.2

Make a leaflet for people with a physical disability that tells them about the person-centred approach and why it may help them.

2.1 Conditions that cause physical disability

There are many reasons for a person to have a physical disability.

Some physical disability may be present when a person is born; this type of disability is called **congenital**. An example of congenital disability is spina bifida and this condition is caused when the baby's spinal cord does not develop properly.

Disability can also be caused by **accidents** which damage the body; damage can be to the body parts, such as arms or legs. Road accidents are the biggest cause of this type of physical disability.

Brain injuries can also cause physical disability. This happens if the part of the brain which controls movement is damaged. Brain injuries like this can sometimes happen during birth but most often happen later on in life. Cerebral palsy can occur when the parts of the brain which control movement are starved of oxygen. This can be during birth or because of an illness that stops oxygen getting to the brain.

Illness from viruses and bacteria can cause physical disability by damaging the body systems that control movement. Meningitis can cause the tissues in the fingers and toes to become diseased and die, which sometimes means that affected parts of the body have to be removed to stop the disease spreading.

Some physical disability is **genetic**, this means that one or both parents have passed on a gene that caused disease or disability. An example of a genetic physical disability is muscular dystrophy. This means that a child's muscles get weaker over time and the child stops being able to walk or is not able to move around as well as they used to.

Assessment task 2.1

Complete the chart below showing some examples of physical disability. Give a short description of the disability and state whether the disability is congenital/genetic or most likely caused by accident or illness.

Physical disability	Description	Congenital/ genetic Or caused by accident/illness
Muscular dystrophy	Muscles get weaker over time and movement becomes more difficult	Genetic
Cerebral palsy		Congenital
Spinal cord injury		Accident
Spina bifida		
Amputation		Accident/illness
Arthritis		

Task!

Research on the internet other causes of physical disability.

3.1 Factors that have a disabling effect on an individual

There are many factors that can have a disabling effect on an individual.

Environment

The **environment** can have a very disabling effect on a person with a physical disability if care is not taken to look at the changes needed to make it safe and accessible to everyone. For example, if a group of teenagers decide to go to listen to live music, and one of the teenagers is a wheelchair-user but the building does not have wheelchair access, that person will not be able to go with their friends. This would make that person feel left out and not part of the group.

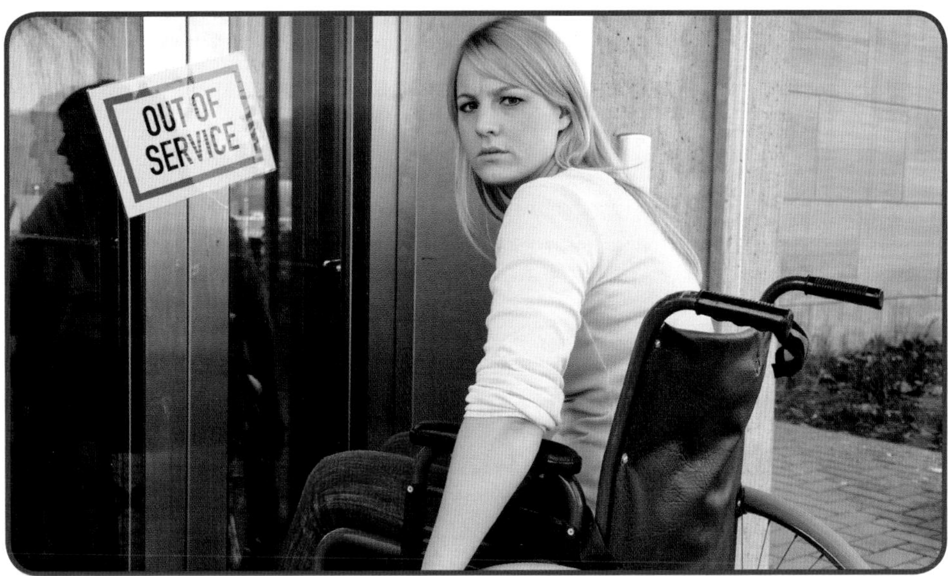

Figure 14.1

Attitudes and beliefs

Discrimination happens when the attitudes and beliefs towards people with physical disability are not positive. This can happen when others do not see the person with a physical disability as a person, like themselves, with feelings, wishes and opinions. Sometimes people feel uncomfortable around a person with physical disability. This might not be because they are thinking unkind things, but because they do not understand disability so they do not know how to behave.

Culture

Some cultures are not very understanding of people with physical disability. If a culture does not understand about physical disability, poor attitudes and unkind behaviour towards people with disability are not questioned or challenged. These types of cultures do not understand the importance of including people with physical disability in their society; this can make the person with a disability feel that they are not part of normal society.

3.2 Give examples of how to challenge discriminatory attitudes

It is important to challenge discriminatory attitudes because a person with a physical disability is a person first, with feelings, needs and wishes. If a person with a physical disability feels discriminated against or not fully included in society because of the attitudes of others, this could leave them feeling sad, lonely, depressed and perhaps angry.

When working in health, social care and childcare, it is important to be a good role model and treat people with disability with kindness and respect. By treating people with a physical disability respectfully, others who are not so understanding will see how to behave and learn the right way to treat people.

If you notice any discriminatory behaviour or feel the attitudes of others are discriminatory it is important to carefully challenge this, perhaps by asking the person why they have behaved in this way and telling them why it is wrong.

3.3 The effects that having a physical disability can have on an individual's day-to-day life

Having a physical disability can have lots of effects on a person's day-to-day life and these can include:

- difficulty getting into and around buildings safely and easily
- having to deal with discriminatory attitudes of others
- tiredness, because of the extra physical effort needed to move around
- problems using equipment such as pens, mobile phones, kitchen utensils, machinery, computers
- travelling during busy times, e.g. busy pavements, crowded trains or buses
- the side-effects of some medicines, such as tiredness or feeling unwell.

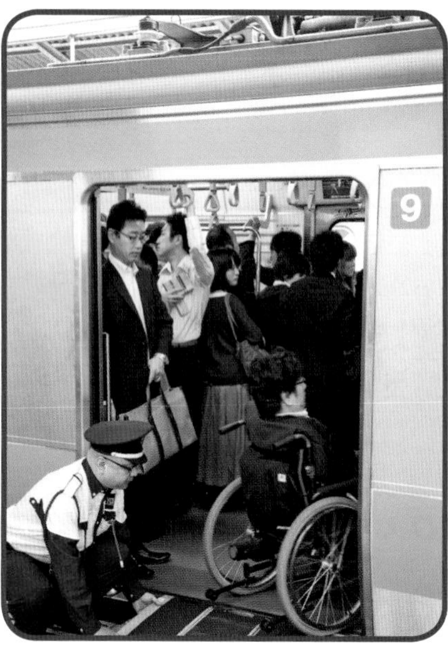

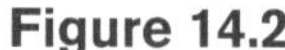
Figure 14.2

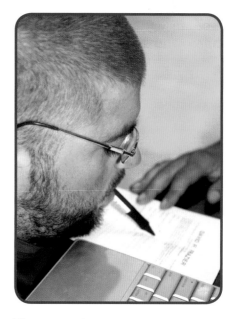

Figure 14.3

Assessment task 3.1 3.2 3.3

Make a poster for school children explaining how **culture**, **environment**, **attitudes** and **beliefs** can have a disabling effect on an individual.

Give some examples of how to challenge discriminatory attitudes.

On the poster, explain the effects that having a physical disability can have on an individual's day-to-day life.

3.4 How individuals can be in control of their care needs

People with a disability may feel that they do not have the same choices or control over their lives as non-disabled people. To allow people with a disability to have equal opportunities, it is important to allow them to make choices about what happens to them. Being at the centre of making decisions about their own care allows a person to feel in control. Ways this can happen are shown in Figure 14.4:

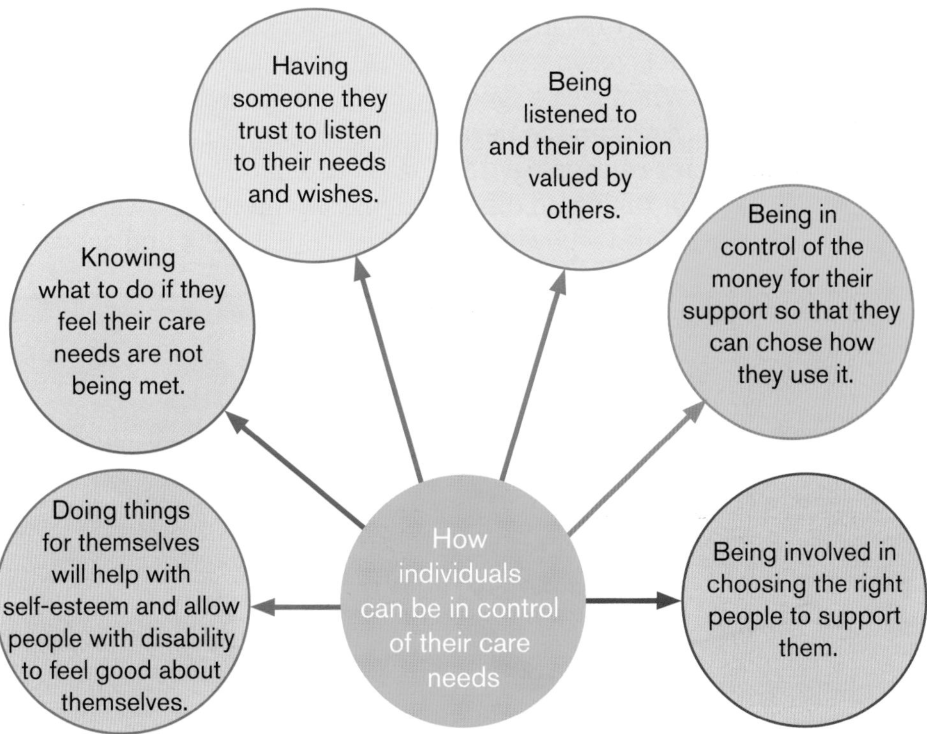

Figure 14.4 How individuals can be in control of their care needs

3.5 The importance of promoting independence for individuals with physical disability

Everyone likes to be independent and in control of their own lives and this is exactly the same for a person with a physical disability.

Having support to live independently is very important for a person with a physical disability. One reason is that when a person can be independent and meet their own care needs, they may have more **self-respect** and there is less opportunity for abuse to take place.

By not always having to ask others for help, people with a physical disability may **feel more confident** and **better about managing their disability**.

By being independent, a person with a physical disability can perform day-to-day tasks in the way they want to do them and when they want to do them. This will make them **feel in control**.

3.6 Ways to promote the inclusion of individuals with physical disability in society

There are many ways to promote inclusion of people with physical disability in society. Pictures in magazines and books, images on the internet and on the television now show positive images of people with physical disability. When we see good images, we are more likely to see the positive side rather than the negative side of something. For example, when we see pictures of people with a physical disability taking part in sports activities or taking on difficult physical challenges, we stop thinking that people with a physical disability cannot be fit and active.

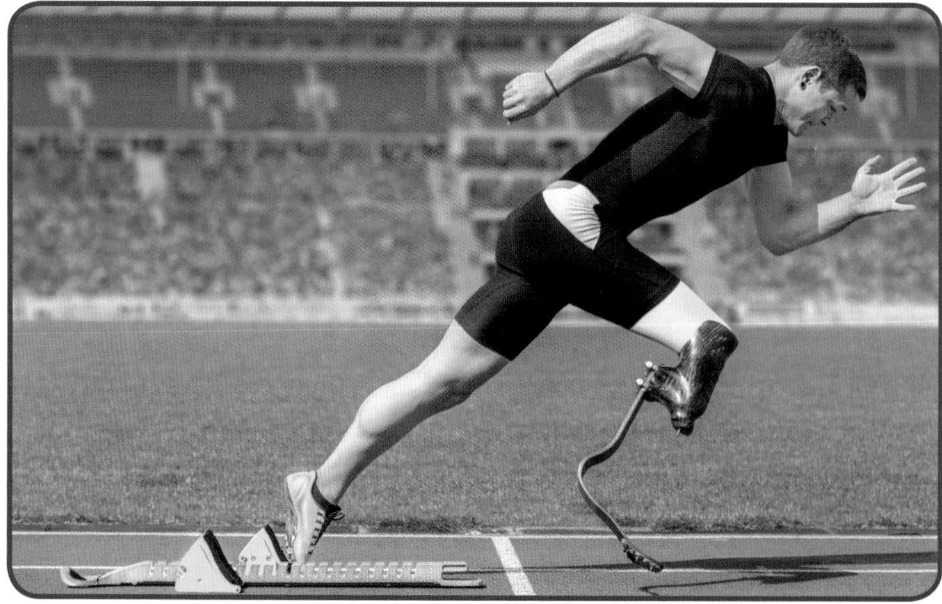

Figure 14.5 A sprint runner with a prosthetic leg

Since the Equality Act 2010, shops and public places such as the cinema, sports centres and cafes must do everything possible to make these places safe and easy for people with physical disability to get around.

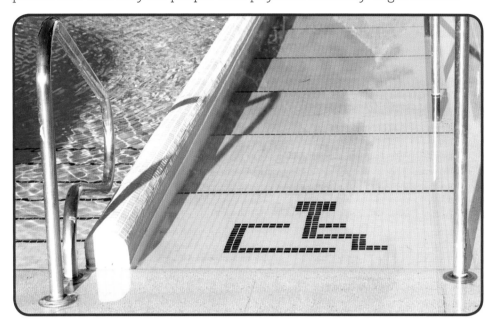

Figure 14.6 Wheelchair access to the pool

Assessment task 3.4 3.5 3.6

Make an information leaflet about physical disability. In the leaflet, describe how people with physical disability can be in control of their care needs.

Write about the importance of promoting independence for individuals with physical disability.

Include information on ways to promote the inclusion of individuals with physical disability in society.

Summary

In this unit you have learned that:

- It is important to recognise and value children, young people and adults with a physical disability.
- There are many causes of physical disability.
- There are many challenges of living with a physical disability.
- Discriminatory attitudes must be challenged.
- It is important to promote inclusion and independence for individuals with physical disability.

Chapter 15

Intro Op 1.8 Introduction to mental health

What you will learn in this unit

- The importance of recognising and valuing individuals with mental health problems.
- How to use a person-centred approach when working with individuals with mental health problems.
- Types and causes of mental health problems.
- The importance of effective communication with individuals who have mental health problems.

Important words

Mental health – Well-being

Mental Capacity Act – Law made to help protect people

1.1 Why it is important to recognise and value an individual with mental health problems as a person first

It is very important to see an individual with mental health problems as a person with feelings and wishes first, rather than focusing on the mental health problems.

It is important to value the person first for many reasons. One reason is that there is a law called the Mental Capacity Act which says that adults with mental health problems should be allowed to make as many decisions as they can for themselves.

A person with mental health problems may feel out of control or feel that no one is listening to them, so it is important

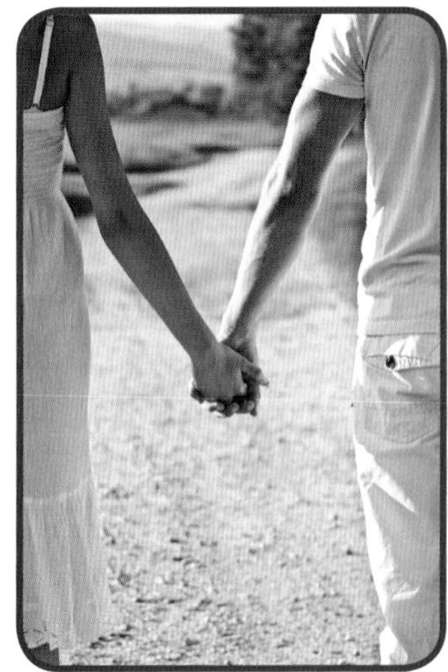

Figure 15.1

that they feel both listened to and in control of what is happening to them.

By valuing the person, not the mental health problem first, the needs of the person can be more easily understood.

When supporting a person with mental health problems, it is important to find out about the person's needs, wishes, likes and dislikes. This is important because everyone has different ideas about what they need and want, and these wishes can be taken into account when looking for the best ways to support the person.

1.2 How to use a person-centred approach when working with individuals with mental health problems

In using a person-centred approach, care workers or health professionals should have a good understanding of the way the person with mental health problems feels and behaves. Care workers should also find out about the person's wishes, needs, likes and dislikes by asking the right questions and listening carefully to their answers.

Care workers may need to get information about the person with mental health problems from other places, such as personal information records or by talking to family and friends. Confidentiality rules should always be followed to keep the person with mental health problems and the care workers safe.

Often people with mental health problems feel very worried or anxious about what is happening to them. The person-centred approach means that care workers need to understand these fears and worries and offer the right support.

Assessment task 1.1 1.2

Write an information leaflet for somebody new to working with people with mental health problems.

- Say why it is important to recognise and value individuals with mental health problems as people first.
- Give examples of how to use a person-centred approach when working with individuals with mental health problems.

2.1 Factors that affect mental health

Factors that affect mental health include:

- **Emotional factors** – This is when an individual feels very emotional, perhaps because something has gone wrong in their lives, they have had a bad experience or they have suffered the loss of someone close to them.
- **Social factors** – This is when an individual feels that they have no friends or they feel left out or all alone. This could be caused by being unemployed or not having enough money to join in any social activities.
- **Psychological factors** – This is when someone has a fear or is coping with trauma such as abuse, or they may have a phobia, for example, being afraid to leave the house.
- **Biochemical factors** – This is when chemicals in the brain change how a person thinks and feels.
- **Genetic factors** – This is about the information in our cells (DNA) that we get from our parents, which affects the way we look, think and behave.
- **Physical factors** – This is when an individual has a disability that makes them feel different, or is worried about how they look and how others might see them.

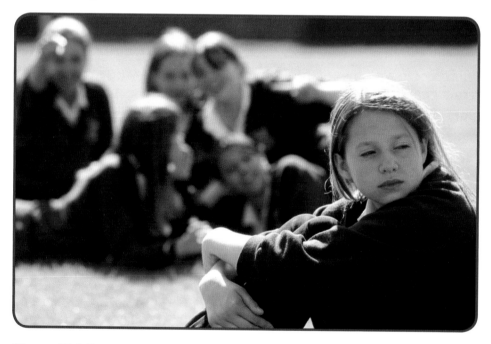

Figure 15.2 Feeling left out may affect an individual's mental health

2.2 Examples of different mental health problems

There are a wide range of mental health problems that can affect an individual and these can include:

Depression – This can affect an individual's mood; they may feel sad or lonely. They may not feel good about themselves. Sometimes an individual with depression may not want to carry out their usual routine, for example, will not want to get out of bed in the morning, or will not want to spend time with their friends.

Anxiety – This can make an individual look or feel scared; sometimes individuals may have panic attacks, feel very nervous or not be able to sleep well.

Self-harm –This is when an individual cuts, hurts or injures themselves on purpose.

Eating disorders – This sometimes includes overeating, cutting out food groups, or not eating enough food to stay healthy.

Stress – This can involve feeling worried, anxious or tense. An individual who is stressed may not be able to sleep well, and their eating habits might change, for example, over-eating or not feeling able to eat.

Bi-polar disorder – A person's moods change between high and low; for example, sometimes being over-excited or at other times feeling very sad and unhappy. Sometimes an individual with bi-polar disorder will behave normally and at other times their behaviour will seem very strange.

Schizophrenia – When an individual imagines that characters or voices that are in their head are real. They may think the characters are talking to them and telling them to do things. Sometimes an individual with schizophrenia will think the voices and characters in their head can harm them.

Assessment task 2.1 2.2

In the leaflet you are writing for health workers:

- Give information about factors that affect mental health.
- Write down four examples of mental health problems.

3.1 The benefits of effective communication on the lives of individuals with mental health problems

It is very important to communicate well with people who have mental health problems as this could make the difference between a person feeling supported and listened to or feeling isolated and alone.

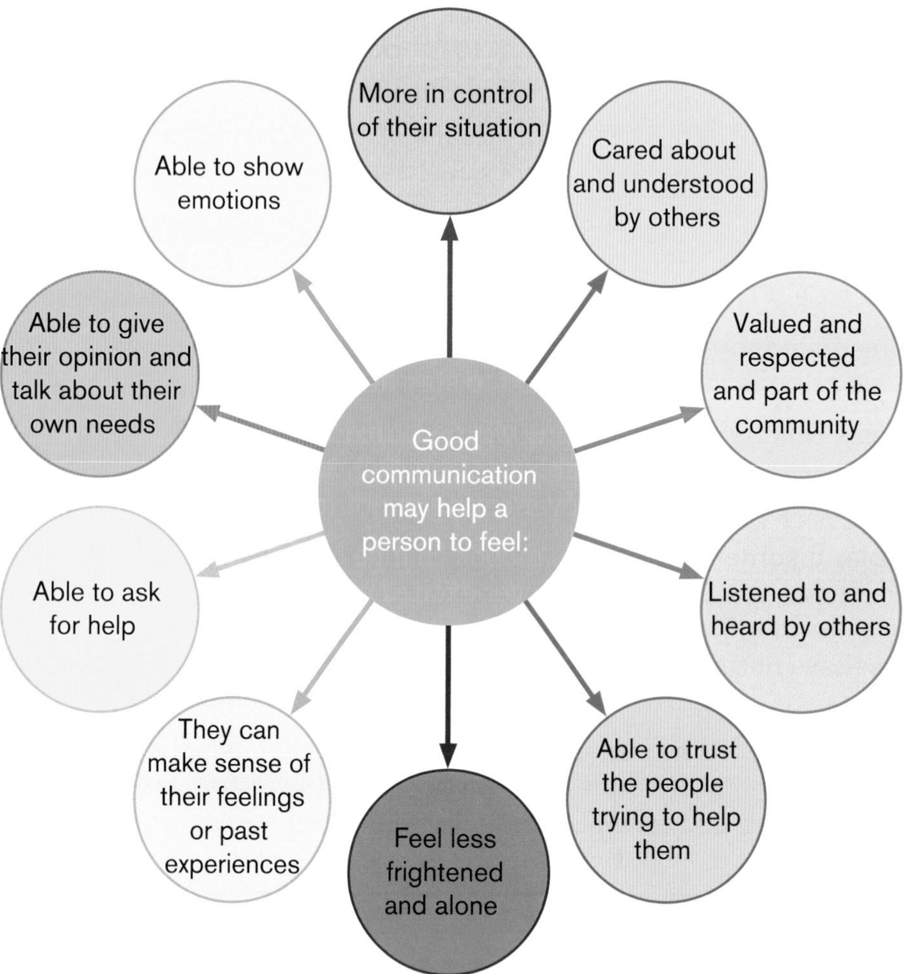

Figure 15.3 The benefits of effective communication on the lives of individuals with mental health problems

3.2 The importance of using active listening skills with individuals who have mental health problems

Active listening is important as this is the main way to find out information about a person with mental health problems. Active listening happens when the professional listens very carefully to what is being said and is not distracted by other things around them. Active listening should take place in a quiet space with no background noise, away from other people.

Active listening helps by giving a person time to tell you about how they feel, what they need and what is happening to them in their lives.

Active listening can be difficult as we may not always listen carefully to what others are saying, because we are thinking about our own opinions or what we need to say next. When we listen actively we need to focus on what is being said and also make sure that we have good eye contact and positive body language that shows the person we are listening carefully and we are interested in what they are saying.

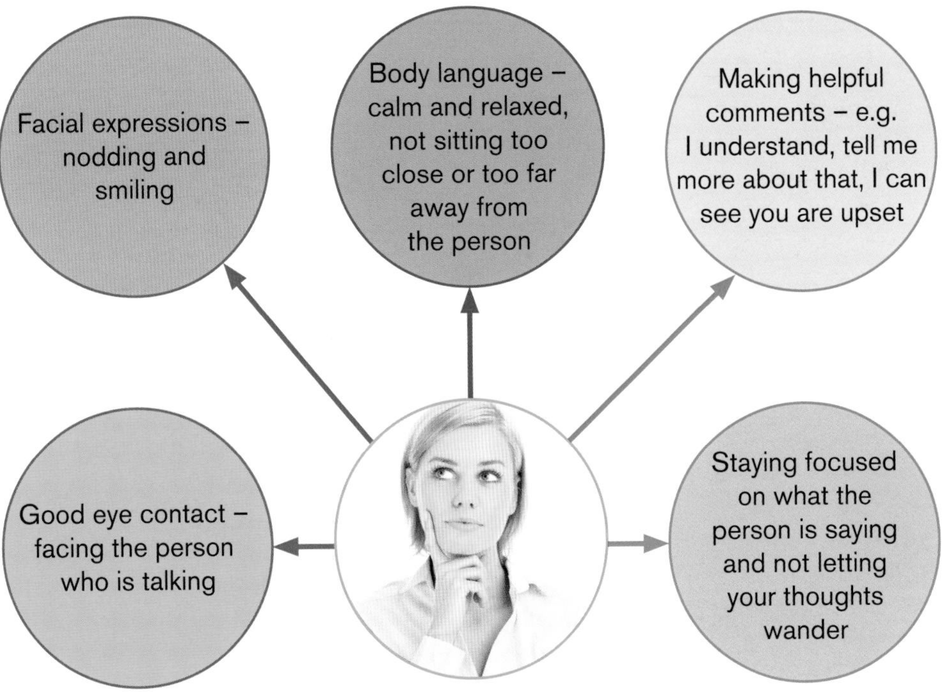

Figure 15.4 Active listening

Assessment task 3.1 2.2

In the leaflet include information about:

- the benefits of effective communication
- the importance of using active listening.

Summary

In this unit you have learned that:

- It is important to recognise and value individuals with mental health problems.
- A person-centred approach should be used when working with individuals with mental health problems.
- There are different types and causes of mental health problems.
- It is important to use effective communication with individuals who have mental health problems.

Chapter 16

Intro Op 1.9 Introduction to dementia

What you will learn in this unit

- Why it is important to recognise and value an individual with dementia as a person first.
- The person-centred approach.
- What is meant by dementia and the main causes of dementia.
- The effects of dementia on families and carers.
- The benefits of effective communication in the lives of individuals with dementia.
- How memory loss affects the use of spoken language in an individual with dementia.
- Techniques that can be used to facilitate communication with an individual with dementia.

Important word

Dementia – When the brain becomes damaged, causing a person to have problems such as not remembering things, not thinking clearly or even losing the ability to speak

1.1 The importance of recognising and valuing an individual with dementia as a person first

The person-centred approach sees the person with dementia as an important individual who has their own interests, opinions, likes and dislikes. Not every person with dementia will need the same type of care and the person-centred approach puts the needs of the individual first.

Health care workers using the person-centred approach find out about the person's individual needs and interests when deciding how to care for them. Individuals should always be treated with dignity and respect.

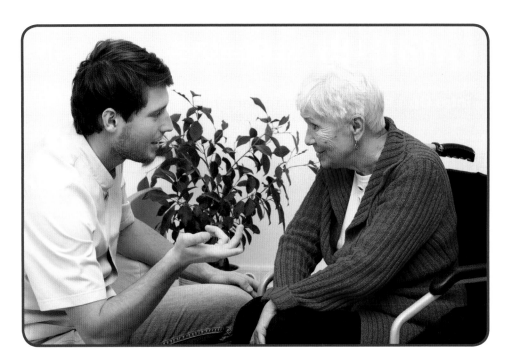

Figure 16.1 The person-centred approach puts the needs of the individual first

1.2 How to use a person-centred approach when working with individuals with dementia

This staff member should have a clear idea of the life history, routines and interests of a person with dementia. Although an individual with dementia may not be able to take care of themselves safely, it is important to give the person safe choices, such as what clothes they would like to wear, if they would like to take part in activities or where they like to sit in a room.

To use the person-centred approach, care workers need to learn about the life history of a person with dementia so that workers are able to talk to the person about their earlier life, or to provide activities that may bring back happy memories of times or places they enjoyed when they were younger. If the person with dementia can do particular things for themselves, they should be encouraged to continue to do so as it will help to keep them active.

Often people with dementia feel worried or anxious about what is happening to them. The person-centred approach also means that workers need to understand the fears and worries that the person with dementia might have and give them the right support.

Assessment task 1.1 1.2

Outline why it is important to recognise and value an individual with dementia as a person first, giving examples of how to use a person-centred approach when working with individuals with dementia.

2.1 What is meant by dementia?

Dementia is a word used to describe a slow loss of memory and thinking skills. This happens because cells in the brain stop working properly. The parts of the brain that are usually affected are the parts that control how we think, remember and communicate.

2.2 Examples of the causes of dementia

There is still a lot of information for doctors and scientists to discover and learn about dementia, but there are four main causes of dementia.

Alzheimer's disease	Scientists have found that Alzheimer's disease happens when **proteins build up in the brain** and they attach themselves to cells. When this happens, the part of the brain that makes new memories stops working first.
Vascular dementia	Vascular dementia is caused when the **blood flow to the brain is not good enough**. Blood carries oxygen to the brain and without it, brain cells can die. This causes the brain to stop working properly and affects memory, language and attention span.
Fronto-temporal dementia	This is a disease that causes some **parts of the brain to shrink** and get smaller. This usually affects the front of the brain that controls behaviour, emotions, decision making, and language.
Dementia with Lewy bodies	Lewy bodies dementia is similar to Alzheimer's because proteins build up in cells in the brain. **Nerve cells are affected by Lewy bodies** in parts of the brain that control thinking, memory and movement.

Table 16.1 Examples of the causes of dementia

2.3 The effects of dementia on families and carers

Having a family member with dementia can have an effect on all members of the family. Some of the most common feelings family members may have are **guilt**, **grief**, **sadness** and **anger**.

Some family members may feel embarrassed by the strange things the person with dementia says or does, and then they feel guilty for **feeling embarrassed** by the person who they love and care about.

People with dementia can sometimes become difficult to manage or they may become angry and aggressive; and if this causes a family member to shout or **lose patience** with the dementia sufferer, they may feel very guilty for shouting or getting cross.

If someone in a family develops dementia, other family members may feel they have lost the person they knew and almost **feel grief** similar to that felt when someone close to them dies. The feeling of grief is for the **loss of the future** that they might have been shared with the dementia sufferer.

Sometimes family members may **feel worried** about how they will cope in the future, worrying about having to put the dementia sufferer in a care home, or they may worry about children in the family seeing the odd behaviour of the dementia sufferer.

It may be that some family members **feel trapped** in their own homes, as they are not able to leave the person with dementia alone at home, so they **stop going out**. The carer may then **lose contact with friends** and begin to **feel lonely**, and perhaps **angry** that this is happening.

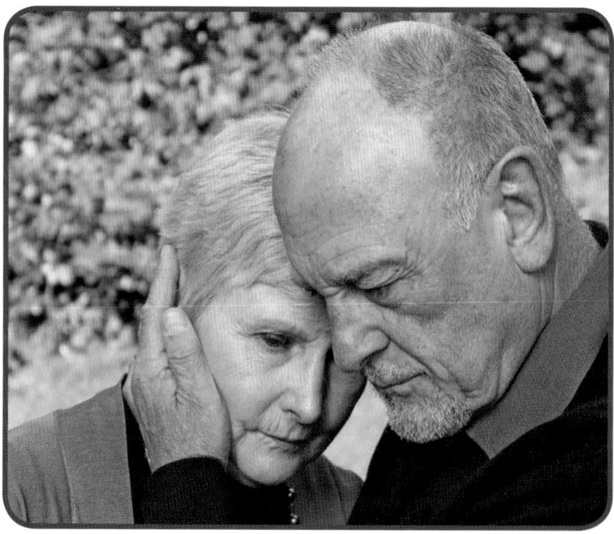

Figure 16.2 The feeling of grief

Assessment task 2.1 2.2 2.3

Produce an information leaflet outlining:

- what is meant by dementia
- giving examples of the causes of dementia.

Include a spider diagram or list of the effects of dementia on families and carers.

3.1 The benefits of effective communication on the lives of individuals with dementia

There are many benefits of effective communication on the lives of individuals with dementia. These include:

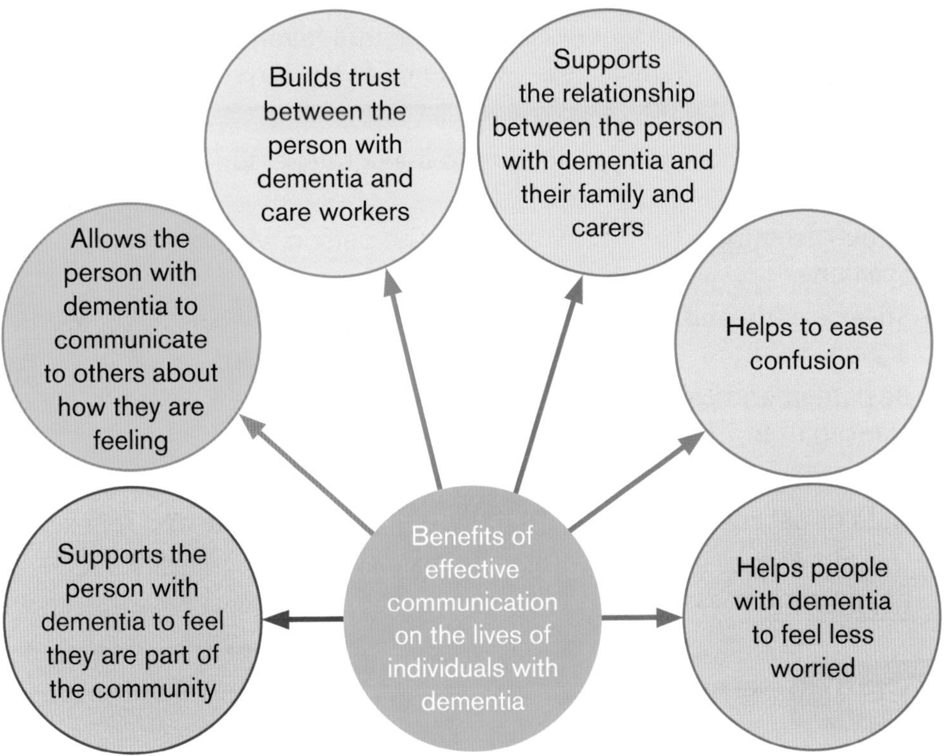

Figure 16.3 The benefits of effective communication on the lives of individuals with dementia

3.2 How memory loss affects the use of spoken language in an individual with dementia

Dementia is an illness which will always get worse over time. The illness slows down the person's ability to think clearly and understand information. This will mean that a person will find it difficult or impossible to remember things such as people's names – even very close family members' names; they will forget dates and places they have been. Dementia will slowly stop the person communicating with other people because they forget the meaning of words needed to make conversation.

3.3 Examples of techniques that can be used to support communication with an individual with dementia

It is important to keep a person with dementia involved in making conversation for as long as it is possible to do so. Ways to encourage communication include:

- Use good eye contact and smiling to make the person feel comfortable.
- Active listening – try not to interrupt the person when they are speaking.
- Speak clearly and slowly so the person has time to think about what is being said.
- Be patient and calm, and give the person time to find the words they want to use.
- Use a friendly tone of voice to reassure the person.
- Hold or pat the person's hand to help them to feel safe and relaxed.
- Use pictures or items from the person's past to help to bring back happy memories.

Task!

Go to **www.nhs.uk/Conditions/dementia-guide/Pages/dementia-and-communication.aspx** and read about the many other ways to communicate with people with dementia.

Assessment task 3.1 3.2 3.3

Identify the benefits of effective communication on the lives of individuals with dementia.

Outline how memory loss affects the use of spoken language in an individual with dementia.

Give examples of techniques that can be used to facilitate communication with an individual with dementia.

Summary

In this unit you have learned:

- why it is important to recognise and value an individual with dementia as a person first
- how to use the person-centred approach
- the meaning of dementia and the main causes of dementia
- how dementia can affect families and carers
- the benefits of effective communication on the lives of individuals with dementia
- how memory loss affects the use of spoken language in an individual with dementia
- techniques that can be used to facilitate communication with an individual with dementia.

Chapter 17

Intro OP 1.11 Introduction to the physical care needs of babies and young children

What you will learn in this unit

- The care needs of babies and young children.
- How to treat babies and young children with respect and sensitivity.
- How to engage babies and young children during physical care routines.
- The principles of toilet training.
- How to provide a safe and hygienic environment for babies and young children.
- How to safely supervise babies and young children.
- What to do to support the well-being of babies and young children.
- The nutritional needs and allergies of young children.

Important words

The Department of Health – This is a Government department that is concerned with the health of the citizens of this country

Physical care routines – A child's day-to-day care needs (skin, hair, teeth, nappy area)

Confidentiality – Only sharing information with people who need to know or can offer help

Nutritional needs – The food a person needs to grow and stay healthy

Allergies – When a person becomes ill from eating or touching a certain food

1.1 Care needs for babies and young children

Skin

A baby's skin can easily be damaged so it is important to use only gentle soaps and shampoos. Baby bath products are made without any harsh chemicals so are just right for cleaning a baby or young child's skin. You should never rub a baby's skin but gently wipe with a clean, wet soft cloth.

You do not need to bath a very young baby every day, but it is important to keep their skin clean and this can be done by top and tailing.

How to top and tail a young baby

- Gently undress the baby, but leave their nappy on.
- Wrap the baby in a soft dry towel.
- Place the baby on the floor on a changing mat.
- Using clean warm water and clean cotton wool, dip a piece of cotton wool in the water and gently clean the baby's face, taking care around the eyes, nose and ears. Use a different piece of cotton wool for each eye.
- Wash the baby's hands and neck area and gently dry them with the towel.
- Unwrap the towel from the baby and take off their nappy. Wash the nappy area, taking care to clean the folds and creases of the skin. Gently dry well with the towel and put on a clean nappy.
- Dress the baby.
- Talk to the baby about what you are doing, smile and give them eye contact – this will help them to relax.

Safety rules 1.1

- **NEVER leave the baby alone near water.**
- **ALWAYS place the baby on the floor on a mat so that they cannot roll off a high surface and get hurt.**
- **NEVER poke cotton buds into the baby's ears or nose as this can cause damage.**

Bath time

It is important to make bath time a relaxing enjoyable time for babies and young children. Young children may enjoy playing with bath toys or helping to wash their own hair. Bath time is a good time to clean a child's teeth.

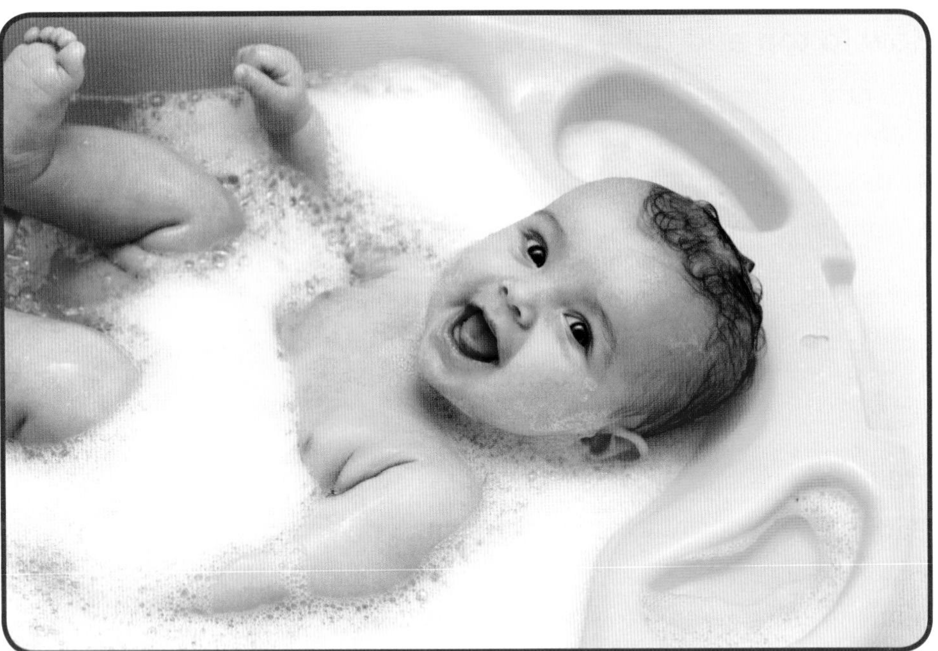

Figure 17.1 Bathing should be relaxing and enjoyable

Bathing a young baby

- Choose a good time to bath a baby, not straight after a feed or when they are hungry or very tired.
- Get everything you need together, including a bath of warm water, a soft cloth, cotton wool, a clean dry towel, bath shampoo and baby bath liquid, a clean nappy and clean clothes.
- Check the temperature of the bath water.
- Clean the baby's face first (read how to do this in the top and tailing section).
- Wrap the baby up using the towel and hold them over the bath to gently wash their hair using a gentle no tears baby shampoo; rinse with the warm water.
- Gently dry the baby's hair with the towel.
- Take off the baby's nappy and wipe away any mess.
- Place the baby in the bath, using one hand to hold their arm to support their head and shoulders with your arm.
- Gently splash the warm water over the child using a clean cloth, taking care to wash in the creases and folds of skin around the arms and legs.

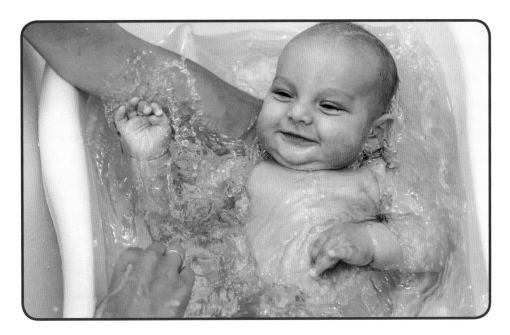

Figure 17.2 How to support a baby in the bath

Bathing a child

Once a child can sit comfortably and safely without the support of an adult, bath time is a much simpler routine. Remember a child will move around much quicker than a young baby so it is important to watch them carefully. Always put cold water into the bath first and add hot water until the water is warm enough. This way of filling the bath should always be used because children can quickly climb into the bath before the bath is ready and hot water could seriously burn a child's skin.

- Get everything ready, including a bath of warm water, soap, hair shampoo, face cloth, clean towels, bath toys, clean clothes and a clean nappy (if the child wears nappies).
- Undress the child and sit them in the bath.
- Talk to the child about what is happening and DO NOT leave the child alone in the bath – not even for a few seconds.
- Wash the child, taking care when cleaning the child's face.
- Wash hair, using a gentle no tears shampoo – the child may like to help. Rinse hair with clean water – using a shower or jug is a good idea.
- Let the child play for a while, but don't let them get too cold.
- Gently lift the child out of the water – take the plug out so that the water drains away.
- Carefully dry the child and dress them. Dry their hair as needed.

Check out this NHS website for a demonstration of bathing a baby:

www.nhs.uk/Conditions/pregnancy-and-baby/Pages/washing-your-baby.aspx#close

Safety rules 1.1

- **ALWAYS** supervise the child around water and never leave them alone in water – not even for a few seconds.
- **ALWAYS** put the cold water into the bath first so that if the child climbs into the bath before you are ready, the water will not burn the child.
- **ALWAYS** check the temperature, either with your elbow or a bath thermometer so that the water is not too hot or too cold (move the water around the bath so that there are no hot areas).
- Make sure the bath water is not too deep.
- **NEVER** take any electrical items such as heaters or music players into the bathroom.

Hair

A young baby does not need to have their hair washed every day. When a baby is being weaned or learning to eat food by themselves, they often get very messy and food gets into their hair, so it is important to wash it more regularly.

It is best to wash a baby or child's hair during bath time, using a mild no tears shampoo. It is important to rinse hair well to get rid of all of the shampoo. Take care with the temperature of the water and always supervise children when they are in the bath.

Hair should be carefully brushed with a soft bristled brush.

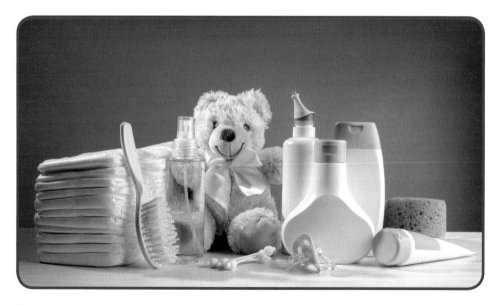

Figure 17.3

Head lice

If a child comes into contact with other children, for example brothers and sisters or friends at nursery, it is important to check their hair regularly for head lice as this is a common problem.

Head lice are tiny, wingless insects that attach themselves to the scalp.

It is very difficult to see head lice and using a fine-toothed lice comb is the best way to find them. Head lice can be treated using special lotions or by wet combing using conditioner and a lice comb. Wet combing done every two days for about 14 days should get rid of the lice.

Further information can be found on the following NHS web page:
www.nhs.uk/conditions/Head-lice/Pages/Introduction.aspx

Teeth

A young child will get 20 first teeth which are called milk teeth and the first tooth cuts through the gums at around six months of age. Some babies will cut their teeth without many problems, but other babies have signs such as:

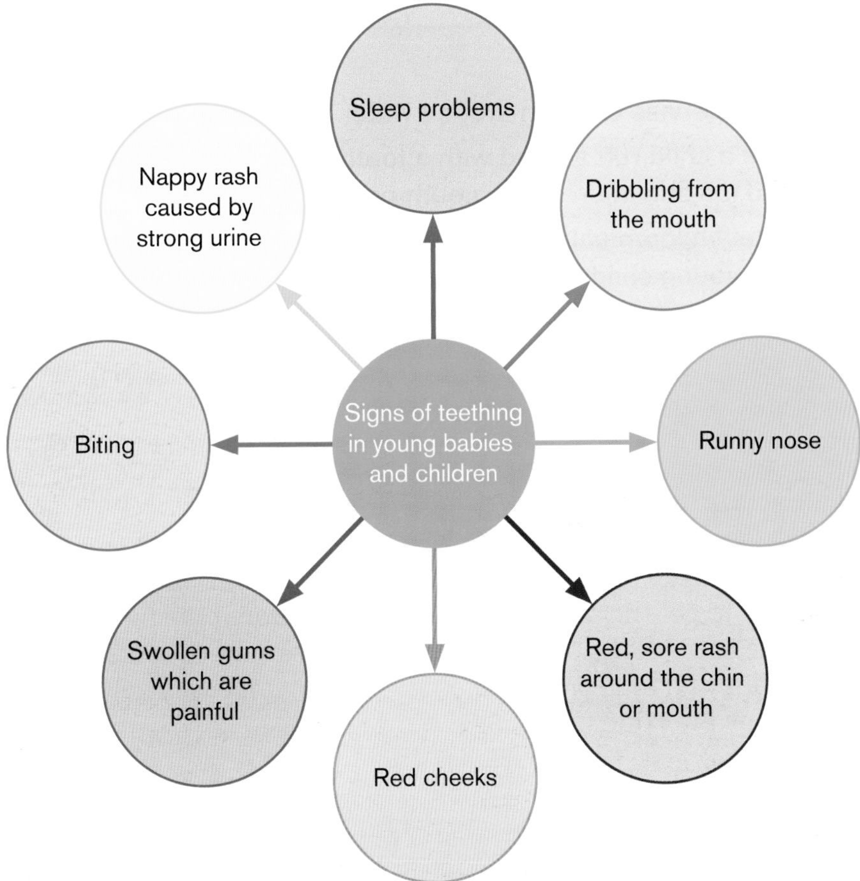

Figure 17.4 Signs of teething in young babies and children

Care of teeth

- It is important to start cleaning a young child's teeth, twice a day, as soon as the first tooth cuts through the gums.
- Teeth cleaning should happen every morning and every evening to help to keep teeth clean and healthy (bath time is a good time to brush a child's teeth).
- Start by doing all the brushing for the young child but, as the child gets older, let them have a go first. By the time the child is about eight years old they should be able to brush their own teeth properly. Use a mirror so that the child can see what they are doing.
- Use a soft toothbrush and mild fluoride toothpaste when brushing children's teeth.
- Brush teeth for two minutes (using an egg timer set for two minutes is a good idea).
- Visit the dentist as soon as the first teeth come through and then follow advice about how often to take the child to see the dentist.
- A low-sugar diet will help to keep teeth healthy and strong.

Safety rules 1.1

- **ALWAYS supervise children around water.**
- **NEVER let a child run around with a toothbrush in their mouth as they could fall and injure their mouth or throat.**
- **DO NOT let children eat toothpaste as too much fluoride can be harmful to young children.**

Nappy area

Always wash your hands before and after changing a baby's nappy.

When caring for a new born baby's nappy area, it is important to use only warm water and cotton wool to clean the nappy area.

It is important to make sure that all soiling is gently removed and care should be taken to get the creases clean and dry before putting a clean nappy on to the baby. Some babies with sensitive skin need to have a very regular nappy changing routine because they can easily get sore skin in the nappy area due to having a wet nappy.

Safety rules 1.1

- **Never leave or turn your back on a baby who is lying on a changing table as they could easily roll off and be seriously injured.**
- **Never leave nappy cream and lotions in a place a baby can reach.**
- **Always put dirty nappies in the outside bin.**

The following NHS website has some further useful information:

www.nhs.uk/Conditions/pregnancy-and-baby/pages/nappies.aspx

Task!

You are caring for a baby aged 12 months. Make a list of all the safety rules when changing and bathing the child.

Assessment task 1.1

Using the information you have read in this chapter so far, complete the table below by identifying the physical care needs of babies and young children.

Care of babies and young children	Identify the care needs for each area
Skin	
Hair	
Teeth	
Nappy area	

2.1 How to treat babies and young children with respect and sensitivity during physical care routines

It is important to always treat babies and young children with respect and sensitivity during physical care routines. Treating children with respect and sensitivity will help them to become confident and feel good about themselves.

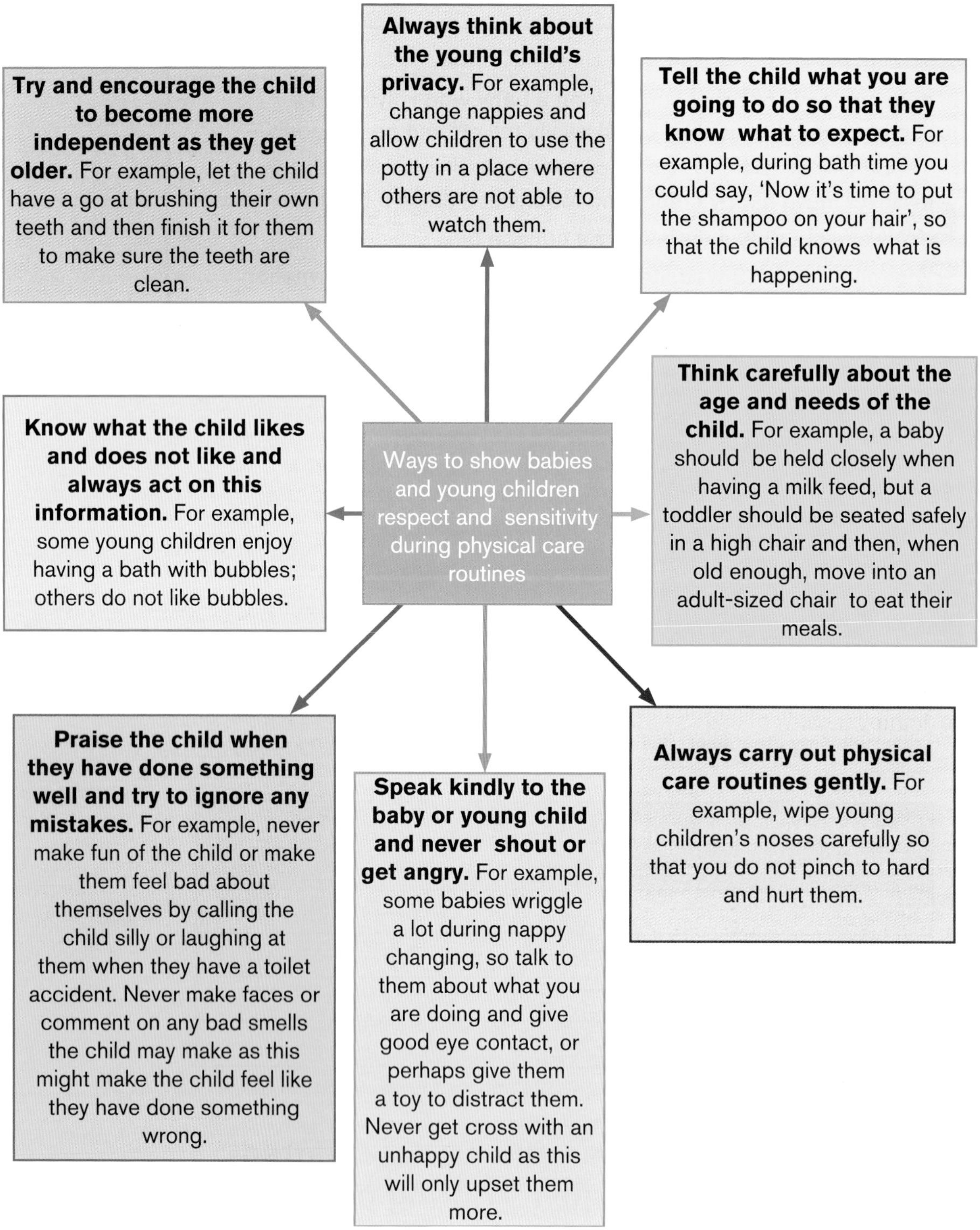

Ways to show babies and young children respect and sensitivity during physical care routines

Try and encourage the child to become more independent as they get older. For example, let the child have a go at brushing their own teeth and then finish it for them to make sure the teeth are clean.

Always think about the young child's privacy. For example, change nappies and allow children to use the potty in a place where others are not able to watch them.

Tell the child what you are going to do so that they know what to expect. For example, during bath time you could say, 'Now it's time to put the shampoo on your hair', so that the child knows what is happening.

Know what the child likes and does not like and always act on this information. For example, some young children enjoy having a bath with bubbles; others do not like bubbles.

Think carefully about the age and needs of the child. For example, a baby should be held closely when having a milk feed, but a toddler should be seated safely in a high chair and then, when old enough, move into an adult-sized chair to eat their meals.

Praise the child when they have done something well and try to ignore any mistakes. For example, never make fun of the child or make them feel bad about themselves by calling the child silly or laughing at them when they have a toilet accident. Never make faces or comment on any bad smells the child may make as this might make the child feel like they have done something wrong.

Speak kindly to the baby or young child and never shout or get angry. For example, some babies wriggle a lot during nappy changing, so talk to them about what you are doing and give good eye contact, or perhaps give them a toy to distract them. Never get cross with an unhappy child as this will only upset them more.

Always carry out physical care routines gently. For example, wipe young children's noses carefully so that you do not pinch to hard and hurt them.

Figure 17.5 Ways to show babies and young children respect and sensitivity during physical care routines

Assessment task 2.1

Make a poster for a health centre outlining ways that babies and young children can be treated with respect and sensitivity during physical care routines.

2.2 Ways of engaging with babies and young children during physical care routines that make the experience enjoyable

- Talking to or singing to a young child during care routines. For example, singing to a baby or young child when changing their nappy.
- Speaking gently and soothingly. For example, when cleaning a child's sore skin saying gently, 'All finished now'.
- Giving the baby or young child eye contact and smiling. For example, looking and smiling at a baby when feeding them.
- Knowing the baby or young child's likes. For example, knowing how a baby likes to be held when being given a milk feed,
- Asking if it is ok to do something. For example, asking a young child, 'Can I wipe your nose for you?'
- Encouraging the child to have a go. For example, washing their own face.
- Joining in with the child so it becomes a more enjoyable experience. For example, cleaning your teeth at the same time as the child cleans theirs.

Assessment task 2.2

List all the ways you can think of to join in a care routine to make the experience enjoyable for a young child.

2.3 Principles of toilet training

Becoming toilet trained is an important time for a young child. All young children are very different and it is not always easy to decide when it is the right time to begin toilet training. Most young children will be ready to start toilet training around the age of two years and will feel more comfortable using a potty rather than a normal sized toilet, which may seem very large to a young child.

Signs that a young child is ready to use a potty

A young child should never be forced to use the potty before they are ready. Young children will only be able to use a potty correctly when their bladder and bowel have properly developed. Some signs that a child may be ready to start potty training include:

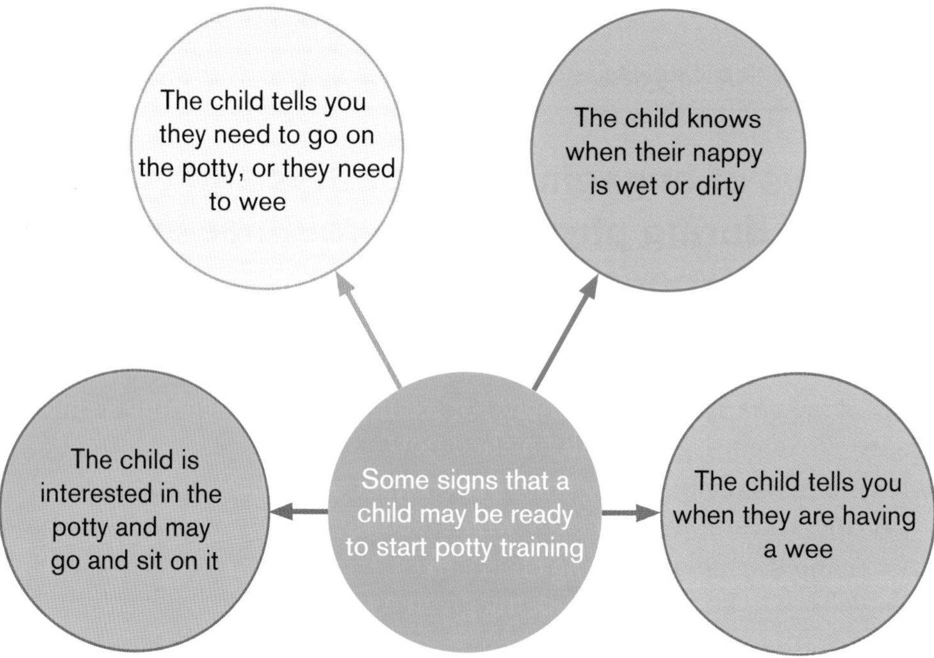

Figure 17.6 Some signs that a child may be ready to start potty training

How to start potty training

- Leave a potty out somewhere that the child can see it and can get to it quickly.

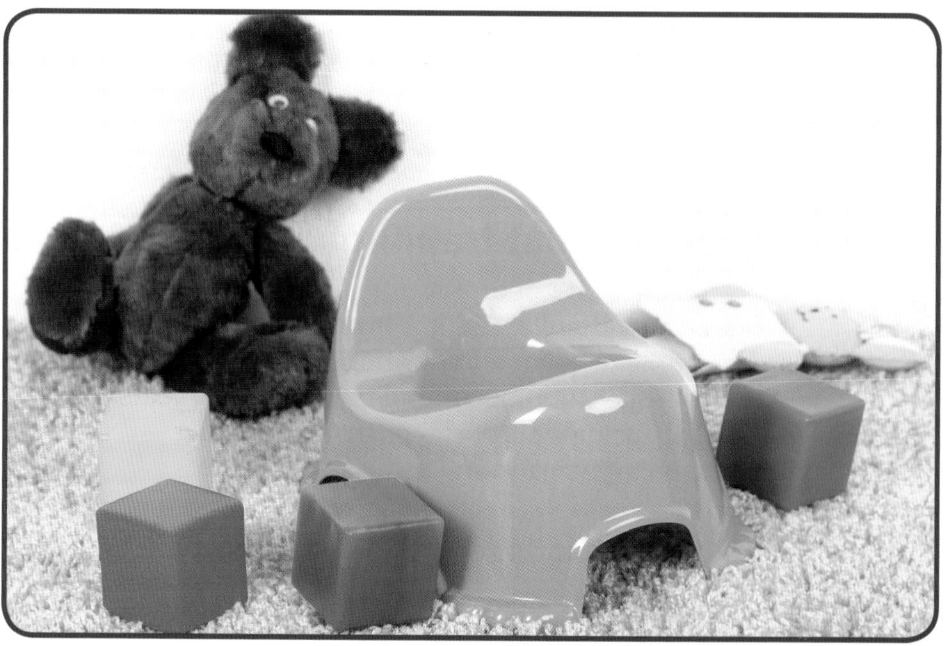

Figure 17.7 A potty in an easily accessible place

- It might help to have another potty beside the main toilet so that the child understands toileting routines.
- If the child has a dirty nappy at around the same time every day, take their nappy off and have the potty in easy reach.
- If the child is upset about sitting on a potty, just put the nappy back on and wait a few more weeks before trying again. Never force a child to sit on a potty as this will upset them and will not help them to become toilet trained.
- If the child lets you know they need to wee, offer them the potty. If the child does not make it on to the potty in time or has an accident, wipe up the spill quickly and do not make a big fuss, because if the child thinks you are annoyed with them they may not want to try again.
- The child will feel very pleased with themselves when they use the potty correctly. It is important to praise them by telling them they have done well.
- Always wash the contents of the potty down the toilet straight away and clean the potty ready to use again.

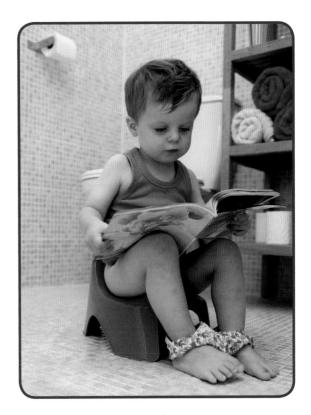

Figure 17.8 A potty beside the main toilet

Task!

- List three signs that a young child is ready to start toilet training.

3.1 What to do if you are concerned about the well-being of babies and young children

When someone is worried about the well-being of babies and young children there are important steps to take to help the child. It is important to be confidential, that means that the concerns are not talked about to anyone apart from the setting supervisor, police or professionals from support organisations.

Firstly, if you see anything that concerns you, it is important to write down the facts; this will include the times, dates and what it is you have seen or heard. This information should then be passed to your supervisor if you work in a setting, or the child's health care professional, such as a health visitor, doctor or social worker. This information must not be discussed or shared with anyone other than the professionals dealing with the situation.

Task!

Discuss in groups the reasons why it is important to maintain confidentiality when there are concerns about the well-being of a child. What might happen if you do not maintain confidentially?

4.1 The nutritional needs of babies

The Department of Health recommends that, where possible, new mothers breastfeed their babies for the first six months of a baby's life. This is because breast milk contains exactly the right amount of calories needed for energy and the right amount of nutrients to help the baby to develop and grow. Breast milk also contains antibodies from the mother which help to protect the baby from illness and diseases.

Scientists who have researched breast milk say that babies who are breastfed do not have as many upset tummies or infections as bottle-fed babies because of the antibodies in breast milk.

Although breastfeeding is the best nutrition for a young baby, some mothers choose to bottle-feed their babies. Babies who are bottle-fed will have formula milk which has nutrients which are as close to breast milk as possible.

Weaning

When a baby gets to around six months of age, milk alone no longer provides all the nutrients and energy needed for healthy growth and development, so the baby will need to be weaned on to solid foods. Weaning begins by offering the baby small teaspoons of baby rice mixed with their usual milk and over time a wider range of foods are added to the diet. To begin with, the weaning foods need to be very smooth and easy to swallow, but slowly the food can be more lumpy and by the time the baby is a toddler they will have teeth and be able to chew and enjoy finger foods such as toast and carrot sticks. By the time the child is around three years of age, they usually enjoy most of the same foods that adults eat.

4.1 4.2 The nutritional needs of young children

(See Unit PWCS 07 for supporting material.)

The nutrients needed by babies and young children are shown in the figure below.

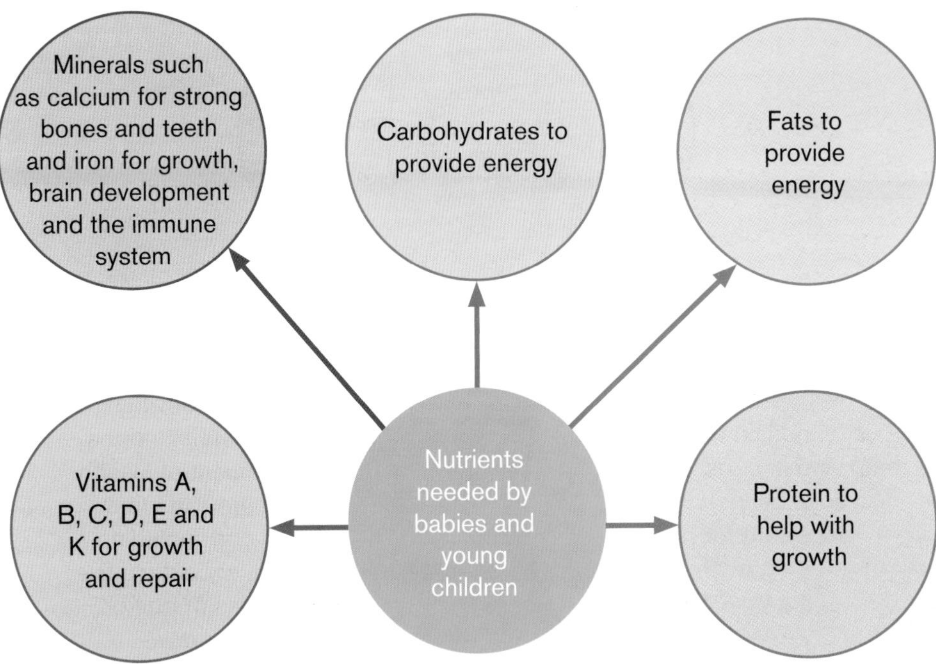

Figure 17.9 Nutrients needed by babies and young children

Which foods contain nutrients?

Milk and dairy foods contain fats for energy and calcium which is needed for teeth and bone growth.

Carbohydrates are found in breakfast cereals, bread, rice and pasta.

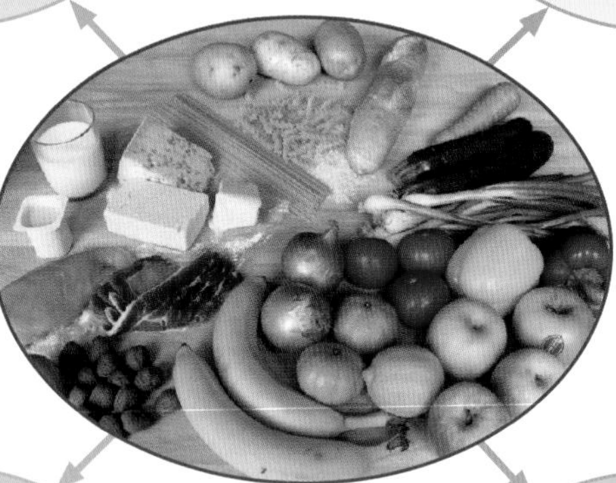

Protein is found in meat and fish and also in eggs and pulses (like soya beans). Protein is important for healthy growth.

Fruit and vegetables contain lots of vitamins and minerals and the Department of Health recommends that everyone, including children, should eat five portions of fruit or veg per day.

Figure 17.10 Which foods contain nutrients?

4.3 Healthy balanced meals for young children

This eatwell plate shows how much of each food type is needed for a healthy diet. The picture shows that the largest part of the diet should come from fruit, vegetables and carbohydrates such as potatoes and pasta. Milk and dairy products should be eaten every day, along with foods high in protein such as fish or meat.

The eatwell plate

Use the eatwell plate to help you get the balance right. It shows how much of what you eat should come from each food group.

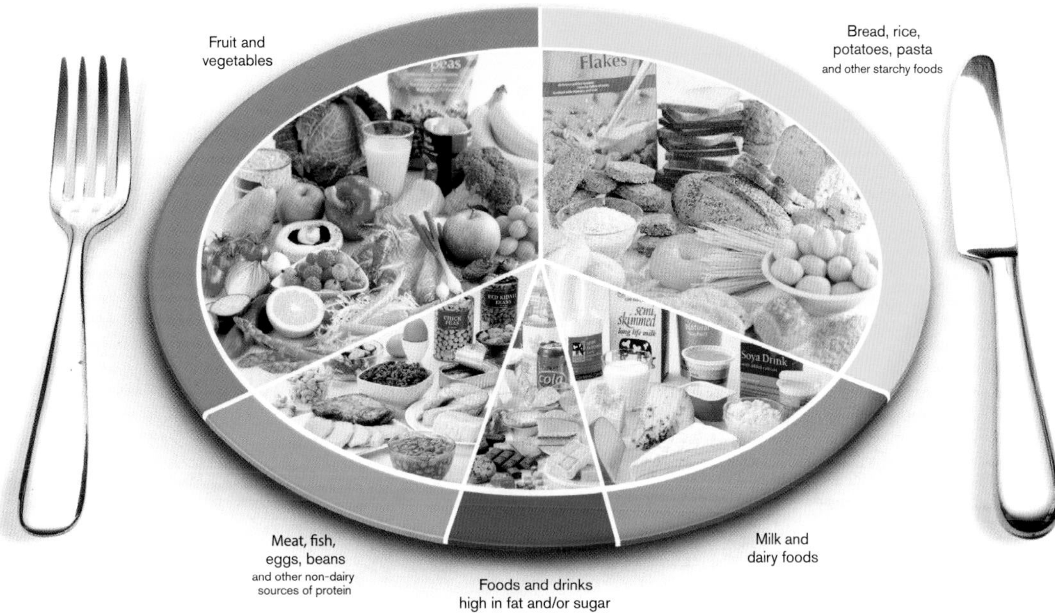

Public Health England in association with the Welsh Government, the Scottish Government and the Food Standards Agency in Northern Ireland

Figure 17.11 The eatwell plate

Source: **www.nhs.uk/Livewell/Goodfood/Pages/eatwell-plate.aspx**

Young children can sometimes be fussy eaters, but it is important that they eat a well-balanced diet that supports healthy growth and development. Food that is very high in fat and/or sugar, such as sweets and crisps, should only be given to children as an occasional treat and should not be given instead of other more healthy foods.

Assessment task 4.2 4.3

Looking at the 'eatwell plate' to get the information about which types of foods are needed in a balanced diet, plan a breakfast, lunch and dinner for a young child, making sure they will get all the nutrients they require for healthy growth and development.

4.4 Nutritional allergies

Some babies and young children become ill when they eat certain foods. These are called nutritional allergies. A mild allergy to a food might cause a young child to have a rash, runny nose, tummy pain or diarrhoea. A doctor can test a child for allergies and the best way to care for a baby or child with a mild allergy is to try and avoid giving the food that causes the problems.

Only a few babies and children have very serious nutritional allergies which cause them to be dangerously ill if they eat certain foods. Eating foods that they are seriously allergic to can cause babies and young children to wheeze or cough, their mouths and tongues can swell so that it is difficult to breathe, and they may collapse or go into shock, which can be life-threatening. Babies and children who have a serious allergy to foods will usually have medication from the doctor or hospital that they can be given if needed. The child should then be taken straight to hospital for treatment.

Foods that may cause allergy are shown in the figure below.

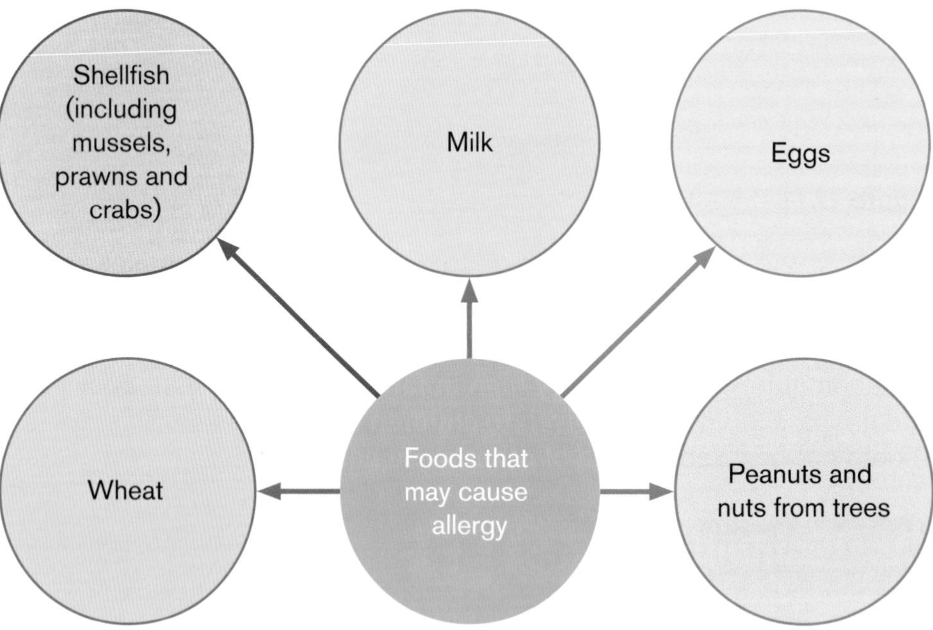

Figure 17.12 Foods that may cause allergy

Summary

In this unit you have learned that:

- Babies and young children have a range of physical care needs.
- Babies and young children should always be treated with respect and sensitivity.
- Physical care routines can be made more enjoyable by engaging with the baby or young child.
- Following the principles of toilet training is important.
- A safe and hygienic environment is very important when caring for babies and young children.
- Babies and young children need constant supervision to keep them safe.
- There are steps to follow when there is a concern about the well-being of a baby or young child.
- Young children have nutritional needs that can be met through having a balanced diet.
- It is important to know which foods to avoid when feeding babies and young children.

Chapter 18

Intro Op 1.12 Introduction to the development of children and young people through play

What you will learn in this unit

- How play supports children and young people's development and well-being.
- The difference between adult-led play and child-centred play.
- How environments can support inclusive and stimulating play.
- Activities that support inclusive and stimulating play.

Important words

Adult-led play – Play activities that are planned and run by adults

Child-centred play – Play that is started and led by children themselves

Inclusive play – Play activities that all children and young people can join in with

Stimulating play – Play that is interesting and enjoyable

Well-being – Feeling comfortable and happy

1.1 How play supports children and young people's development and well-being

Play is a very important part of children's learning and development. It is through play that children use their senses and, while having fun, they can be creative and can also learn about the world around them. When children and young people play, they are developing new skills and practising skills they have already learned. When children and young people play together, they are learning to work as a team and to co-operate with each other.

When playing happily with others, children and young people will feel accepted in the group, which will support their well-being. Being outdoors and having exercise while playing will also support feelings of well-being.

When playing outdoors, children and young people are able to learn about risk and challenge. This is when they have to decide for themselves if something is safe to do, for example, jumping off a climbing frame. If the child falls when they land, they will learn that they have climbed too high to jump safely, but if they land safely, they will know that they have good physical skills and will feel proud of themselves.

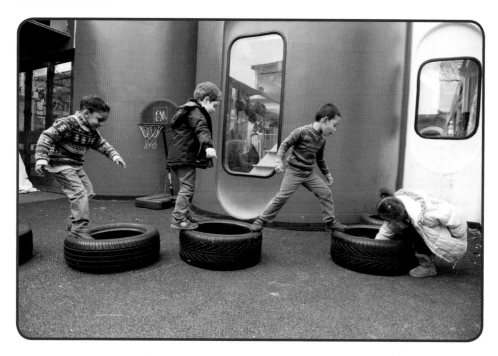

Figure 18.1 Children playing outdoors

Assessment task 1.1

Make an information poster about play.

Write down some reasons why play helps children's development and well-being.

1.2 The difference between adult-led play and child-centred play

Child-centred play is when the child makes choices about what activities they join in with or what toys they play with. The child makes up the rules and decides how to play and how long to play. During child-centred play, the child is in control and adults will only get involved if the child is not playing safely.

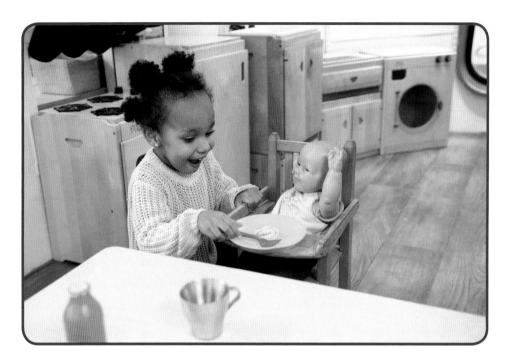

Figure 18.2 Child-centred play

Adult-led play is when the adult plans the activities and the adult provides the equipment that they would like the child to use. The adult usually has a good idea of what the child should be doing and will support the child to be successful.

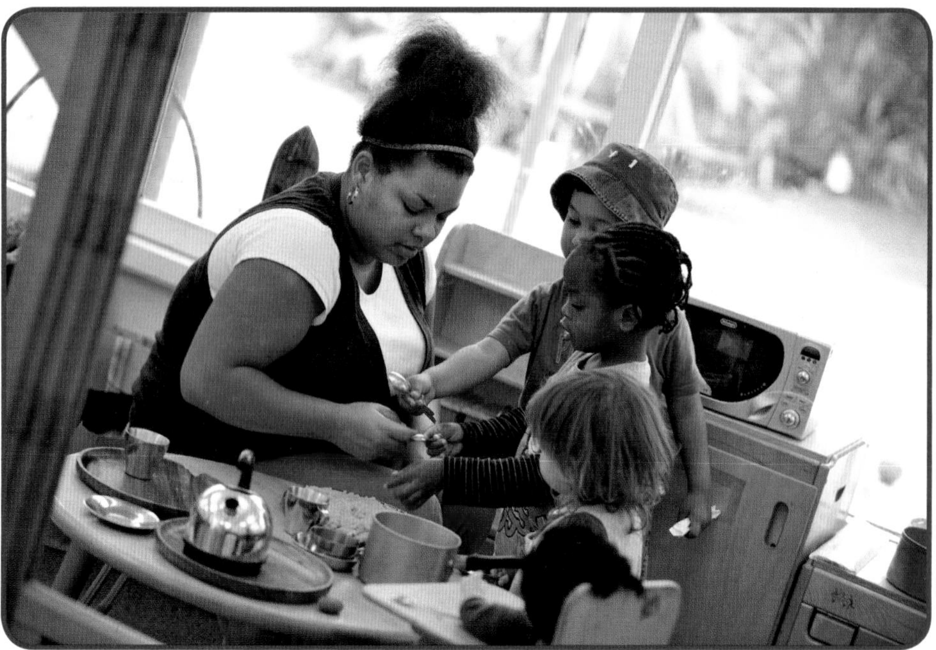

Figure 18.3 Adult-led play

Assessment task 1.2

On the information poster about play, write down the difference between adult-led and child-centred play.

2.1 Inclusive and stimulating play

To provide inclusive and stimulating play in a setting, care workers should understand the needs, interests, likes and dislikes of all children and young people in the group.

Inclusive and stimulating play is when all children and young people in the group can enjoy taking part because the activities are planned around their interests and meet all of their needs.

2.2 Environments that support inclusive and stimulating play

Both indoor and outdoor settings can support inclusive and stimulating play. It is important that there is a mixture of child-centred and adult-led play, so that children can enjoy activities that are planned by the adult and activities they choose for themselves.

A wide range of activities should be available for children and young people, so that they are given a choice of things that they enjoy and are able to do. It is also very important to have activities that the children and young people have not tried before so that they are able to have new experiences and develop new skills.

The care workers or nursery workers must think about the individual needs of children when they set out activities, toys and equipment so that all children can take part. Some children need to have special equipment to allow them to take part in an activity; for example, a child who is left handed will need to have left-handed scissors when they are doing a cutting and sticking activity. If there is a wheelchair user or a young person has sight impairment, the furniture will need to be set out in a way that makes it easiest for them to move around safely.

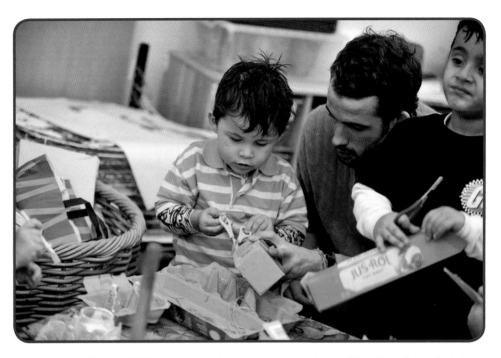

Figure 18.4 Some children need to have special equipment to allow them to take part in an activity

Care workers are also an important part of the setting so they should offer encouragement, praise the children and young people and give them the right amount of help when they ask for it.

Assessment task 2.1 2.2

On the information poster about play write down:

- the meaning of 'inclusive and stimulating play'
- what makes a setting 'inclusive and stimulating'.

2.3 Activities that promote inclusive and stimulating play

There are many types of play activities that allow all children to have fun and learn new skills.

These can include:

- **Creative play**. This is where children and young people use things like crayons, paint, paper, glue, or other materials to be creative. It also includes activities like playdough, sand play, junk modelling and cutting and sticking. It is important to remember that left-handed scissors should be available for children who are left handed.

- **Physical play**. This is where children and young people can enjoy using their physical skills such as running, jumping, catching and throwing. Physical play can be enjoyed in groups, for example tag or hide and seek, and team games such as football or netball can help children to understand team work and develop their physical skills.
- **Imaginative play**. This is where children and young people pretend to be someone or somewhere else. Children and young people do not always need to have any equipment to enjoy imaginative play; for example, young children who are pretending that they are lions or tigers will just get down on the floor and make roaring noises.

Equipment and props, like a home corner in a setting or an outside den, can help children to use their imagination. A young child may pretend that the cardboard box they are sitting in is a car, or a group of children may dress up as pirates and pretend the box is a boat on the high seas.

Assessment task 2.3

Make a list of other creative, physical and imaginative activities that all children and young people could take part in and enjoy.

Summary

In this unit you have learned that:

- Play supports children and young people's development and well-being.
- There is a difference between adult-led play and child-centred play.
- Environments can support inclusive and stimulating play.
- Activities support inclusive and stimulating play.

Glossary

Abuse – To be treated in a damaging way by one or more people

Adult-led play – Play activities that are planned and run by adults

Allergies – When a person becomes ill from eating or touching a certain food

Antioxidant – Antioxidants work to reverse the damage that pollution has on the body

Assessing risk – Seeing things that might be a danger to someone

Assist – Help

Balanced diet – Daily food that has the right amount of nutrients for health and growth

Barrier – Something that gets in a person's way and may stop them from doing something

Child-centred play – Play that is started and led by children themselves

Circumstances or life events – Situations or experiences in a person's life

Communication methods – Ways to communicate

Confidentiality – Only sharing information with people who need to know or can offer help

Contribute to helping an individual stay healthy – Help a person to stay healthy

Contributes – Helps to support

COSHH – The law linking to the Control of Substances that are Hazardous to Health

Dehydrated – Dried out and thirsty

Dependent – Needing the help and support of others

Discriminatory attitudes – The poor attitude and behaviour people show towards others with disability

Discriminatory attitudes and behaviour – When someone judges another person or group of people because of the way they look, how they speak, the music they listen to or the clothes they choose to wear

Emotional and social well-being – Happiness in yourself and as part of a group (society)

Employee – Workers

Employer – Someone or an organisation that pays workers for their work

Employment – A job that you are paid to do

Equality – Making sure all people are treated fairly

Evacuate – Leave a building or area safely

Expected pattern of development – This is the order in which most people develop

Factors – Negative or positive things that may have happened

First aider – Someone with a first aid qualification

Formal communication – When information is shared in a professional way. Slang words are not used.

Guidance and standards – Rules and guidelines that should be followed

Harm – Injury or hurt caused to someone

Hinder – Stop

Inclusion – Being part of something, being included, or making sure everyone can be included

Inclusive play – Play activities that all children and young children can join in with

Independent – Not always needing the help and support of others

Inform individuals – Let people know

Informal communication – Speaking with friends

Legislation – Laws or rules which must be followed

Leisure activities – Interests or hobbies that people can enjoy

Life event – Something that has happened to a person that has affected their life, such as serious illness or loss of a family member

Lifestyle – Way of life

Mental Capacity Act – Law made to help protect people

Mental health – Well-being

Neglect – This happens when someone is not looked after or cared for properly

Non-verbal communication – Ways to communicate without speaking

Nutrients – Are found in food and do an important job to keep the body healthy

Nutritional needs – The food a person needs to grow and stay healthy

Pathway – A timeline

Person-centred practice – Listening to a person and meeting their individual needs in the way that is best for them

Physical barrier – When someone is stopped from taking part in an activity because the environment and/or equipment does not meet their individual needs

Physical care routines – A child's day-to-day care needs (skin, hair, teeth, nappy area)

Prevent – Try to stop something from happening

Principle and values – The main beliefs and ideas of an organisation

Procedures – Steps to take when doing a task

Promoting independence – Encouraging someone to find ways to do things for themselves

Recommended daily fluid intake – The amount of water that experts say we should drink everyday

Releases – Frees

Respecting and valuing – To show care and consideration of others' views and opinions

Safe disposal – To throw away safely

Safeguarding – Protecting children and adults from harm, abuse or neglect

Safety control – Things that can be done to reduce the risk of injury

Self-esteem – Feeling good about yourself and having confidence

Service provision – These are services that are available for people to use

Service user – Someone who uses the service

Social activities – Free time that people can enjoy with others

Social barrier – The way people are treated by others which can stop them being included or taking part in an activity

Stimulating play – Play that is interesting and enjoyable

Support organisations – Organisations such as Childline, NSPCC, Action on Elder Abuse which work to protect children and adults

Support relationships – Enjoy friendships and meet new people

Teamwork – This is when people work well together

The Department of Health – This is a Government department that is concerned with the health of the citizens of this country

Verbal communication – Speaking and listening

Vulnerable person – Someone who could easily be hurt through attack, neglect or unkindness

Well-being – Feeling comfortable and happy, also health and happiness

Index